Yoni Massage

Awakening
Female
Sexual Energy

Michaela Riedl

Translated from the German
by Nikolas Win Myint

Destiny Books
Rochester, Vermont

Destiny Books
One Park Street
Rochester, Vermont 05767
www.DestinyBooks.com

Destiny Books is a division of Inner Traditions International

Originally published in Germany under the title *Yoni Massage: Entdecke die Quellen weiblicher Liebeslust* by Hans-Nietsch-Verlag
First U.S. edition published in 2009 by Destiny Books

Photographs by Bernd Eidenmüller with assistance from Frank Fleuchaus
Photograph on page 8 by Monika Neumann.
Illustrations by Ella Gluck except as noted below.
Illustrations on page 16 from Jane Patterson et al., *Frauenkörper neu gesshen* (Berlin: Orlanda Frauenverlag, 1997), 38, 39.
Illustrations on page 37 from Sabine zur Nieden, *Weibliche Ejakulation* (Giessen, Germany: Psychosocial Publishers, 2004), 13, 15.

Library of Congress Cataloging-in-Publication Data
Riedl, Michaela.
   [Yoni Massage. English]
   Yoni massage : awakening female sexual energy / Michaela Riedl ; translated from the German by Nikolas Win Myint.
      p. cm.
   Includes bibliographical references and index.
   ISBN 978-1-59477-274-0 (pbk.)
   1. Women—Sexual behavior. I. Title.
HQ29.R54 2009
306.7082—dc22
                                                                      2008048960

Printed and bound in the United States by Lake Book Manufacturing

10   9   8   7   6   5   4   3   2   1

Text design and layout by Virginia Scott Bowman
This book was typeset in Garamond Premiere Pro, with Baskerville, Trajan Pro, Atlas Greeting, and Gil Sans as display typefaces

Dedicated to my mother, Roswitha Riedl, and my father, Friedrich Riedl, in gratitude for their love and respect;

My friend Gitta Arntzen, with whom I lead AnandaWave, in gratitude for the realization of a shared vision;

My teacher Maraya, in gratitude for lighting the spiritual spark in my life.

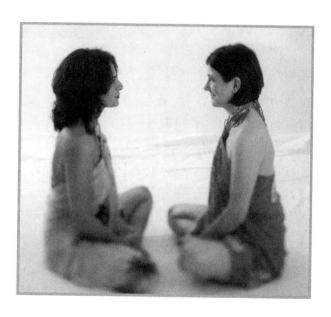

Contents

Preface

The female mystery has beguiled us since time began. Because a large part of female sexuality takes place hidden from view, it leaves much room for fear and speculation. It also leaves room, however, for fantasies, desires, and hopes. Many women and men that I encounter have a serious wish to learn more about female sexuality—holistically and in depth—but they often feel helpless and inadequate to do so.

Early in my own life, I felt an impulse to learn more about my yoni, and a desire to get in touch with the feelings that were associated with it. I was curious about my desire and joy, and about the emotions and moods that sometimes blocked the realization of that joy. However, it soon became painfully clear to me that our society hardly offers opportunities to approach this topic in a respectful and appropriate way. Yet how are we to be in touch with the beauty and essence of our sexuality when we have such a limited space in which to experience it? A yoni cannot reveal its secrets or its overwhelming joy by following narrow norms; it can reach full bloom only when we experience all its depths.

Female sexuality is an indefinite space that becomes bigger, more intense, and more pleasurable the more we experience it in a protected space. Respect and attention are keys to appreciating the many facets of the yoni and receiving its gifts of fulfillment and joy.

My many questions and hunger for experience led me to take part in a tantric yoga course from 1995 to 1997. It was there that I learned for the first time about yoni massage, an extensive and intensive massage of the female genital area. The yoni massage work had lasting effects on my sexual experiences and also taught me much about true sexuality. I became aware of how closely my yoni was linked to my whole being—to my inner growth, my happiness, and my desire for life. I have encountered nothing since then that has affected me on so many levels: on a physical level as a source of health and vitality, on an emotional level through intensive dealings with my feelings, and on a spiritual level through the experience of my spiritual breadth, which is part of the heart-opening effects of yoni massage.

While I had been searching up until then for meaningful work, this experience immediately made clear to me what my calling was. Since then, I have explored the yoni in many ways—by myself, and together with other people who share my urge to learn more about the healing dimensions and strength of our sexuality. In 1997, I met the shaman teacher Maraya Haenen, who deeply affected my life and thinking. With Maraya's guidance I immersed myself in the spiritual aspects of sexuality and tantra, which became the foundations of this book.

Since 1997, I have offered seminars and massages for people who want to learn more about themselves, about sensual touch, and about the power of sexuality. Along with my business partner Gitta Arntzen and many others, I created a healing center called AnandaWave—Space for Spiritual Experience. AnandaWave offers massages, seminars, and counseling that provide women and men with opportunities to encounter sexuality in a healing way. For me, sexuality is the most fundamental source of spiritual and physical well-being, which in turn lead to growth and health. My vision is for all people on this earth to recognize the yoni for what it is: the universal lap of woman, from which we all come, and which we should all remember to honor.

Even after years of work, the transformations that happen at AnandaWave continue to touch my heart and make me happy. Within a short period of time, clients begin to open themselves and allow themselves to be touched. When I look people in the eye after a good massage or a good seminar, I see increased depth and empathy, as well as more clarity, loving presence, and profound openness. After massage women often tell me that they have never before been touched so thoroughly and with such undivided attention. Many report that they have previously been very much fixated on reaching climax, which had precluded awareness of anything else: sensations such as the widening of the yoni, emerging feelings, merging with the partner, the opening of the heart, the steadily growing and expanding desire, and the circulation of energy in the body had all been lost. Some women recognize themselves as sexual beings only after their first yoni massage, while others begin to realize that they carry deep wounds in themselves.

It takes many small steps to experience sexuality in a deep and healthy way. I do not believe in one-size-fits-all solutions for problems or for unfulfilled desires. Healing begins with a journey, and we must open ourselves to the process. The yoni massage is one possibility that is important to me personally, since the massage touches the innermost parts of womanhood. It is a small step to a more fulfilled and consciously lived sexuality.

This book is intended to support women in adding more vitality, healing, and desire to their lives, and in opening the way to a new understanding of their femininity. For men, it is an invitation to learn more about the female mystery and to develop a better understanding of it. I sincerely hope that my book offers knowledge and inspiration to its readers, both male and female. I hope that it will provide the seed for valuable and healing experiences and contribute to people experiencing their relationships and sexuality as a source of internal riches. Where love resides, there is no longer space for violence.

WITH SENSUAL GREETINGS,
MICHAELA RIEDL

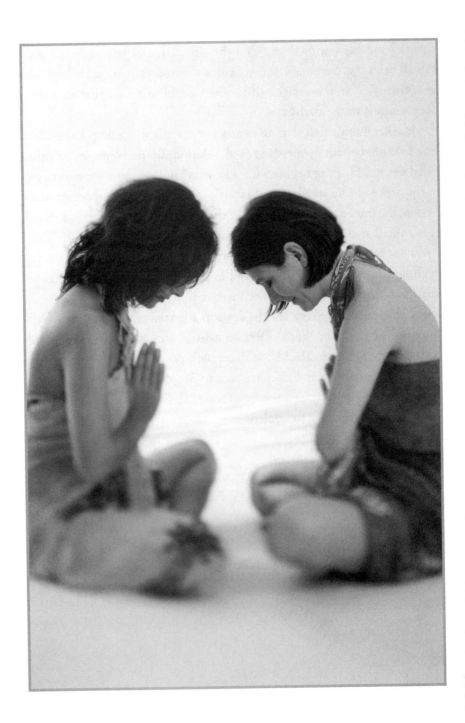

Introduction

A woman who has discovered her sexuality and draws strength from it is radiant, creative, and filled with vitality. She embodies the beauty of life and in turn attracts this beauty like a magnet.

The yoni is the key to discovering this empowering form of sexuality; it opens our innermost core. The word *yoni* comes from the Indian Sanskrit and refers to the entire female genital area, from the external parts of the vulva to the vagina, uterus, and ovaries. I am deeply grateful to have finally discovered a beautiful term for female genitalia, since I never found anything in the German language that even came close to describing the beauty and dignity of women's bodies.

No yoni ever tires of sending new signals as an invitation to us. We are connected to it at the most fundamental level, and we can neither ignore it nor ban it from our lives. Whether we are young or old, seventeen or seventy-seven, whether we are filled with beautiful experiences or lonely or traumatic ones, our yonis always maintain open pathways to our inner selves and will never be entirely closed to us. It is thus unimportant where we are in our sexual experiences when we decide to embark on a journey of discovery to the depths of our yoni.

What we can discover on this journey is the flower of our femininity and the power of our independence. A woman who knows her yoni knows her desires and is able to communicate them clearly. This self-awareness and confidence find expression in all other parts of her life and are transferred to her entire being.

When women are fulfilled and knowing as a result of close contact with our femininity, we are able to build bridges to men. We no longer need to defend our boundaries in a hostile manner, or to wait quietly for a man to fulfill our hidden desires. We ourselves know what we need and can express these needs in a clear and loving way. From my years of leading seminars I know that men are incredibly grateful when they have concrete information and no longer have to search in the dark. When they know exactly what a woman likes, they are usually ready with their whole heart to translate this into respectful, careful, and loving practice.

An important goal of this book is to provide more understanding, knowledge, and new perspectives, which together will create the basis for allowing ourselves to look in a new way at the old injuries that have been created over centuries and passed on through generations. This will enable us to take an active and courageous step forward, into a happier and more self-directed future. With detailed descriptions of yoni massage, I want to offer readers the possibility of approaching the yoni in a practical and sensitive way.

Before going into the individual phases and steps of yoni massage, it is important to look at the many layers of the female genitalia. First, we have to understand where we will find what—what happens when I open the outer labia; where will I find the clitoris pearl with its hood; what do the inner labia cover? Where do I find the urethra? Where is the opening of the vagina and that of the anus, and what exactly lies between the two? These questions may seem obvious to some, but I continue to encounter women who are surprised to learn that urine does not come from the vaginal opening but from the opening of the urethra above it, which is pin-sized and leads to the bladder.

I encounter even more uncertainty and insecurity among women and men when we talk about the innermost point of the female genitalia. Where exactly is the mysterious G-spot? Does it even exist? Where does the vaginal canal end? The vagina itself is not a pipe that is always open and receptive but is made up of the upper and lower vaginal walls, which rest snugly on top of one another and have to be opened carefully before something can be inserted with ease. To know even this much seems very important to me.

Once we are familiar with the external and internal areas of the yoni and know exactly where to find what, we can dare to go a step further:

how do the different parts feel? Women can feel each touch clearly and will notice that the feelings become more intense as the relationship with the yoni becomes closer and more clear. Men have the possibility of letting themselves be guided by a woman, or guided by their own intuition, and thus become ever more aware of female body language.

In this context, it is useful to know that the clitoris is made up not only of the visible small pearl but also has a shaft with two legs—the entire thing has the incredible length of ten centimeters—through which it is present in the entire female genital area. Moreover, the pelvic floor muscles can stimulate the clitoris even without direct contact. Once we know how to use even these little bits of information in a practical way, we can enrich our sexual lives enormously.

To enable men to have an approximate idea of how the individual areas feel to women during stimulation, I've included a section titled "Gender Similarities in Anatomy and Sexuality" (page 32), which lists the parts of women and men that are similar in their sexual reactions. For example, an extensive massage in the area of the G-spot for women feels somewhat like an extensive prostate massage for men.

Many people stop after the discussion of anatomy and don't give much further thought to the subject of sexuality, but the sweetest experience of female sexuality can be found only by leaving the usual paths and diving into the depths of female sensation that are neither visible nor concretely touchable. This world opens itself to us as soon as we close our eyes and direct our attention inside ourselves. When we experience a feeling, for example caused by the stimulation of our clitoris, we can recognize the feeling and either observe it from the outside or actually become the feeling. All of us know the difference between these two. We can be happy about a birthday present and perceive this feeling as happiness, or we can be entirely swept up and thus become the happiness ourselves. Our heart opens up, our breathing deepens, our eyes glow, and when we walk out on the street, we encounter lots of friendly people. The bus driver says a friendly hello, the neighbor does us a favor, and the flower shop gives us a rose as a present. We embody this happiness so much that it affects those around us.

What exactly happens to us in moments like these? And how can we consciously create them? Humans are made up of energy and it is what keeps us alive. We all know people who have too little energy and who seem slow and tired as a result, and we also know people whose overabundant energy drives them to become uncontrollable in daily life. An electric toothbrush works if we give it energy in the form of electricity, and it stops working when the energy source is removed. Slower movements of the brush signal that the battery is close to running out. With people, the situation is very similar.

The energy inside us affects our whole being. Our body, our thoughts, and our consciousness are made up of energy. Body, soul, and feelings form an indivisible whole. They are closely linked to each other through the endocrine system, the central nervous system, and the immune system. We recognize a lack of energy as pain, listlessness, or dullness.

At times our sexuality can bring us into contact with intense feelings, which then have an immediate effect on our body and soul. Knowing this, we can choose to accept our ever-more-intense feelings. We can completely give in to them, using breathing and consciousness to bring the intense energy flow through our bodies, until we reach a point where we have suddenly become one with the feeling. It is in this moment that an infinitely deep and peaceful space opens up. In this space, there is no "I" observing from the outside; we melt and become one with all that exists. For me, this oneness is spirituality.

When we understand how the energy created by sexuality flows through our bodies, we can support and strengthen the process in a number of ways—in particular through our breathing. With the help of particular breathing techniques (see page 75), sexual energy can be spread across the whole body, filling us with health and vitality. When the energy begins to flow, our hearts open and we feel happy, safe, and deeply loved. In this state we feel strong, confident, and alive.

We cannot truly understand this process, however, until it is rooted by experience in each cell of our bodies. Nothing can replace our experiences. The best massage technique in the world is of no use if we forget the love that is needed to heal our hearts and our humanity. This love leads us to new ways of creating respectful interactions with our sexuality.

Because of my tantric yoga experience, I understand yoni massage most completely in the light of tantric philosophy, which builds a bridge between body and soul, and between sexuality and spirituality. Tantra cultivates the senses to the point where we can recognize sexual strength in its full spectrum and use it for our health, spiritual growth, and mental presence.

Thus I always see the practical application of yoni massage as work on consciousness. Experiencing the depths of our sexuality allows us to enter new spaces of consciousness, where we recognize that we are part of a whole with which we are irreversibly linked. We become aware that all of our actions have effects on ourselves and our surroundings. From this recognition, which can be attained only with an open heart, we develop a desire to be responsible in this web of life.

Despite all the knowledge that we can gain about the yoni and yoni massage, the fact remains that we are dealing with a mystery that we should not desecrate by being too analytical or too narrow in our interpretations. It is a world that we can experience most intensely in the enveloping and protecting twilight between consciousness and the subconscious. An analytical light that is too bright desecrates the intimacy that is created when we give ourselves to the process of yoni massage freely and without expectations. In the experience of this spiritual, powerful space, and in the peace that we encounter there, lies the uniqueness of yoni massage.

1

Female Sexuality

I do not search, I find.
Searching, that is starting from existing circumstances,
And wanting to find the known.
Finding, that is the entirely new.
All ways are open, and what is found is unknown.
It is a daring, a holy adventure:
The uncertainty of such risks could in fact only be taken
    by those
Who feel comfortable in uncertainty,
Who in not knowing, and not leading,
Are led,
Are pulled by the destination,
Rather than determining it.

—PABLO PICASSO

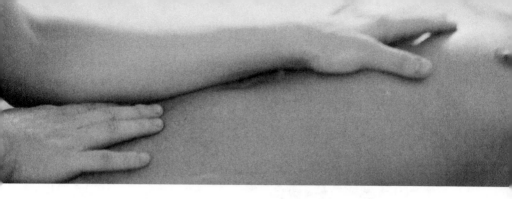

Throughout history, and in different cultures around the world, women have been assigned various roles—sometimes as initiators or love goddesses, at other times as tools of the devil or as playthings of man. Somehow we are consigned to extremes either of beauty and purity or of sin and shame.

In the tantric tradition, women are admired for their power to initiate others, while the yoni is honored as a healing place and residence of the goddess. Each woman is seen as the embodiment of sensuality, as transmitting sexual strength and creativity. This praise of the female goddess and her arts of love is described in Indian works such as the Kama Sutra and the Ananga Ranga, which elevate sexual passion to a spiritual level.

The tantric tradition seeks to connect the worldly and the spiritual. In this context, the union between woman and man is a ritual act of central importance. It is an embodiment of the union of Shiva, the male godly principle, with Shakti, the female godly principle, and a reenactment of their dance that unites the polarities of life.

The Shiva lingam (*lingam* is the Sanskrit word for penis or phallus) and the Shakti yoni are honored throughout India in sculptures that depict a large lingam stone resting in a holy yoni bowl. The Shiva lingam is the embodiment of cosmic creativity and transcendence, while the yoni represents an entrance to the original "holy shrine"—the place where holy conception takes place. Everyday rituals in India involve people placing flowers and offerings on this symbol, and pouring milk, oil, or holy water over it.

In almost all cultures with a strong spiritual foundation, we find traditions that honor women as powerful sexual initiators. Old teachings and writings from Greece, Egypt, Arabia, India, Tibet, and China express these traditions. Chinese literature, for example, contains a number of poetic names for the female genitals, such as "jade gate," "cave of desire," "valley of joy," "ruby-red slit," and others. (However, these traditional

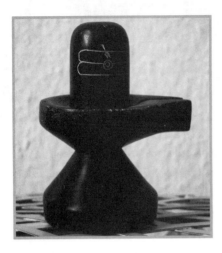

*Fig. 1.1. The Shiva lingam
in a yoni bowl*

writings were written by a small learned elite, and they did not find a concrete way into people's everyday lives. When we look at these same cultures today, we no longer see evidence that they honor female sexuality. On the contrary, the topic of sexuality is taboo in India and many other countries, and women are treated with little respect.)

Christianity, with its negative view of anything related to the flesh, is traditionally unfriendly toward sexuality. This attitude is also reflected in many of our languages, which do not contain any beautiful or loving names for the reproductive organs.

We are confronted with these contradictory extremes—from praise to condemnation—as soon as we begin to deal with female sexuality. When we begin to make contact with our yoni, it is likely that we will encounter this contradiction in ourselves. One participant in one of our seminars about yoni massage described it in this way: "I always feel as if a washerwoman is standing next to me, with her finger raised and commenting on every feeling. Then I am embarrassed about everything and ask myself what I am doing here and whether this is normal. I feel caught, as though I were doing something very bad, even though I know that I am finally opening myself to something that is good for me."

I suppose that each woman finds this contradiction in herself in some way. I know hardly any women who haven't imagined themselves in the role of a whore at some time in their fantasies, even though they are moral in their daily lives. We should thus listen with interest to what these voices inside our heads are saying, because they reflect the contradicting thoughts and feelings that pull at us every day, whether we are conscious of them or not. If we don't confront these feelings in ourselves, we will not be able to engage our sexuality without judgment. Only when we know these thoughts can we begin to deal with them; once the voice inside has said all it wants, we can thank it and return our attention once again to our yoni. We can touch it gently and feel exactly how this feels, in order to enter a dialogue with these feelings. The feelings then come to the foreground, and the judging voice loses its significance. In this way, nobody can make us doubt ourselves, and we can enjoy our sexuality with confidence and control.

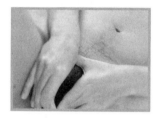

EXPLORING THE YONI

If you would like, you can now take the time to look at your yoni. For this, you will need a mirror. Ask your yoni how it would like to be touched. You can also celebrate the exploration of your yoni together with a partner, as long as you know each other well and trust one another. For this, find a safe, comfortable, and warm room, which you make appealing to yourself. If you wish, you can talk to your partner about your internal dialogues when they take place, but the point is not to appraise, comment, or discuss your thoughts. Whether alone or with a partner, make the exploration of your yoni as joyful and lively as it is sensual and pleasurable.

When you are looking at your yoni in a mirror from a standing or sitting position, you often see little more than a hairy triangle and perhaps further down the clitoris and the Venus lips, or inner labia. I use the term Venus lips instead of labia, since this area for me has nothing to do with shame.*

According to Taoist teachings, our labia contain our fear of opening ourselves, and our desire to hide. Both feelings can be released through

---

*Translator's note: The German author makes this reference to shame because in German the inner labia are called *Schamlippen. Scham* translates as "shame," "modesty," or "bashfulness." In addition, the pubic bone is called the *Schambein,* or shame bone.

massage. Also according to these teachings, the clitoris stores nervousness, mistrust, impatience, and tension. Again, massaging the clitoris can
resolve these blockages.

To explore your yoni, sit down close to or on top of a mirror. You
can use a regular handheld mirror for this or, better yet, a slightly larger
mirror that leaves both your hands free so that you can explore your yoni
with your fingers. If it is your partner's yoni that you wish to explore, ask
her to allow you to look at her yoni.

The Venus mound (mons veneris) is usually hairy and toward the bottom ends in the outer labia, which are also usually covered by hair. The
inner and outer labia form a protective oval that envelops the inner, more
sensitive part of the yoni. The oval formed by the outer labia begins with
the band of the clitoris and ends with its lower tip in the dam that is
called the perineum. The perineum is about one inch long and forms a
bridge to the anus.

A yoni is as unique as a face: in some women, the outer labia may
cover both the clitoris and the inner labia, while in other women, the
outer labia may be flat, leaving the clitoris and inner labia clearly exposed.
Other women may have very long inner labia, while the clitoris is surrounded by the outer labia.

If you gently pull apart the outer labia using the fingers of both hands,
you will be able to more clearly see the clitoris pearl with its tentlike hood.
The sides of this hood end in the two inner labia, either directly or with a
seamlike connection. The inner labia also form an oval, from the hood of
the clitoris to the yoni opening (vagina entrance). A little further up you
can see the opening of the urethra. This opening, through which urine is
excreted, is usually no larger than a pinhead and is easiest to find when
you use one finger to gently pull the yoni opening downward, causing the
upper area to tense slightly. In this way, the opening of the urethra, which
is usually surrounded by folds of skin, becomes more easily visible. It ends
in a short path that leads to the bladder.

The yoni opening is surrounded by a jagged ring, the remains of the
broken hymen. The hymen is a tissue layer that covers the yoni opening,
either partially or entirely, until a woman has sexual intercourse or until
the hymen is broken by other events, such as insertion of a tampon, masturbation, or sports.

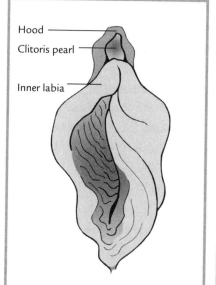

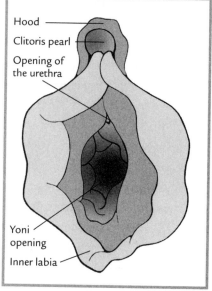

Fig. 1.2. The outer characteristics of the yoni (closed yoni)

Fig. 1.3. The outer characteristics of the yoni (open yoni)

Next, we reach the inner area of the yoni. For this, it is best to use plenty of lubricant and to make sure that your hands are pleasantly warm. People often picture the vagina as a tube that is always open and ready for receiving the lingam. In reality, however, it is usually closed, with the lower and upper vaginal walls resting on top of each other. The yoni first has to be gently opened before it offers its full depth and breadth. Deep breathing, sighing, and moaning facilitate access to the temple of your yoni, or your partner's yoni.

By slowly and carefully inserting one finger, you can explore the inner area of the yoni. It is best to approach this holy place with consideration and empathetic attention. The inner area of the yoni feels completely different in each woman. Usually it is warm, at some spots even hot, and has an uneven surface like a crater. The depth of the yoni can vary from two and a half to ten and a half inches, and the opening in a relaxed normal state can be between one and three inches wide.

The upper area of the vagina is best felt by using your middle finger to slide into the yoni, with your palm facing up. This upper zone is connected directly with the very sensitive urethral sponge, which makes it receptive to sensation and therefore of great importance to sexuality, as we will see later.

Among many women, the lower area of the vagina is far less sensitive. This does not mean it should be ignored, however; the area can store memories of deep psychological injuries, which may present themselves as hard areas, knots, or particularly hot spots. A woman may have difficulty reaching her own lower vaginal area, which is best reached by crouching, then sliding the thumb into the yoni and pressing it slightly downward. If you are exploring the lower vaginal wall of your partner, use your middle finger, with your palm facing down.

If you now insert one—or even better two—fingers deep into the yoni, you can feel the cervix. You may find the cervix either right in the center or slightly above or below the center, as it can bend in different directions. The cervix is surrounded by very subtle spiritual energies, which can be activated through touch. If you no longer have a cervix, you can touch the scar tissue surrounding this area, which will also activate these subtle energies.

Now that we have an overview of all areas of the yoni, we can discuss each area in further detail..

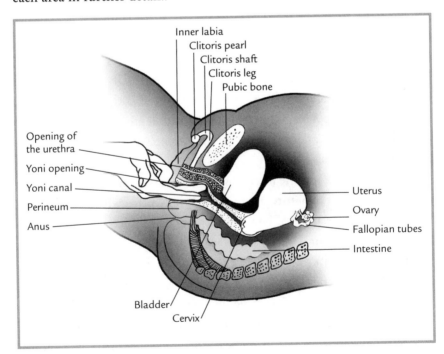

Fig. 1.4. Massaging the upper yoni wall

Venus Lips: The Labia

When we look more closely at the outer labia, we find that they are usually covered by more hair than the inner labia and are less sensitive to touch. They can be very large and meaty, or flat and thin. In some women, the outer labia have a slightly darker color than that of the surrounding skin.

The inner labia are usually not covered by hair and are very sensitive to the touch. The can be very thin and skinlike, but also short, thick, wrinkly, or meaty. In some women, they are much longer than the outer labia, while in others they are tiny and can barely be recognized. The two sides can also have different sizes and/or shapes. Sometimes the inner labia have a pink tone, sometimes they are brown on the outside and red on the inside, or brown-purple, or pink-purple.

The inner sides of the outer and inner labia are smooth and shiny. They are covered densely by oil and sweat glands as well as nerve endings. In the case of sexual excitement, the blood circulation in the outer labia increases, and they turn a glowing red. In my experience, women love to receive a long and extensive massage of the outer and inner labia before the stimulation of the clitoris. Touch on the outer labia is always received with pleasure, even if it does not cause great sexual excitement.

Massage of the inner labia leads to much more intense reactions. Many women experience strong sexual stimulation here, partly due the fact that this massage almost inevitably reaches the clitoris pearl. The inner labia are very sensitive to the touch, so a massage should definitely include plenty of lubricant. Some women may complain of light pain, especially when being massaged on the lower part of the inner labia. This can be caused by uneven stimulation from hands and fingertips, which register very strongly and negatively in this area. You should also make sure not to have any rough edges on your fingers that could scratch the sensitive skin.

℘ *Touching the Labia*

1. Make sure that you or you and your partner are in a protected and lovingly furnished room—if you like, complete with sensual scents, pleasant music, and candlelight.

2. After sufficient preparation, for example a short or long full-body massage (see page 108), or if you are doing this by yourself, after you have

touched your body lovingly, you can begin by applying (unscented) lubricant to your entire yoni.

3. Now lightly pull out the outer labia and touch and massage them slowly with light circling movements from top to bottom. Begin with one side of the labia, then turn to the other. At this point, you are concerned primarily with establishing contact. How do the outer labia feel on your fingers? What do you feel when you touch yourself or are touched there? What thoughts are coming up inside you? What does your internal voice tell you?

4. Enter into a dialogue with yourself or tell your partner exactly what you are feeling at this moment.

5. Whenever a particularly intense emotion rises inside you, recognize it. Take a deep breath and simply allow the feeling. Perhaps you are sad because you realize that your labia have never before received this much attention, and that they have missed this attention and touch. Perhaps you are happy about the touch. Whatever feelings come up, take deep breaths and accept these feelings.

6. Continue with the touch and gentle massage of the inner labia. As you did with the outer labia, pull them out slightly and begin massaging them with light, circling movements from top to bottom, beginning first on one side and then moving to the other. How do the inner labia feel between your thumb and index finger? How are they different from the outer labia? What sensations are you feeling? Simply acknowledge these feelings, without trying to to feel something in particular.

7. Make sure that you have enough time to continue exploring these feelings, and to take a little rest after the massage.

The Clitoris

After this massage, the outer and inner labia are surely awake, with blood circulating freely, which is a good time to enter into deeper contact with the clitoris. When we speak of the clitoris, most people think of the visible and very sensitive clitoris pearl. However, the clitoris is made up of four parts, through which it extends throughout the pelvic floor: the pearl (glans clitoridis), also called the clitoris pearl or tip; the prepuce (praeputium clitoridis), also called the hood or hat; the body (corpus clitoridis), also called the shaft; and the legs (crura clitoridis).[1]

Like much else about the yoni, the clitoris varies widely in its size and shape. The pearl, for example, can have a diameter of between one and fifteen millimeters, meaning it can be tiny or the size of a hazelnut. I once saw a woman with a clitoris the size of a hazelnut and was overwhelmed, since the clitoris pearl is small and hidden in most women, becoming easy to feel only when they are aroused. Sensitivity and sexual stimulation are completely independent from the size and shape of the clitoris, however. Finally, the clitoris pearl is not always entirely round but can be pointed or sometimes even split into two distinct parts.

The length of the clitoris body is between one-half centimeter and four centimeters. This is the area behind the pearl. It is easiest to feel this shaft by rubbing your thumb and index finger from the pearl backward and then forward again. It feels like a round, movable, rubber ring.

The pearl and shaft are partially or entirely covered by the prepuce, or more precisely, the hood. This hood can be long and full or short and covered by skin. The hood serves to protect the sensitive clitoris pearl from being permanently stimulated, even though the pearl is entirely free and curious. For some women, you have to first pull back the hood before you can see the pearl. The legs stretch along the pelvic floor like an inverted "Y" along the clitoris shaft, though they are neither visible nor accessible to the touch. The total length of the legs is around seven and a half centimeters. When we add the length of the legs to the average size of a nonaroused clitoris pearl (half a centimeter) and the average length of the shaft (two centimeters), then the entire clitoris, at ten centimeters (nearly four inches), is significantly larger than most of us assume (see figure 1.5 on page 16).

Almost all muscles in the pelvic floor area cover the clitoris legs, and most are also connected to the sensitive clitoris pearl in one way or another. The two muscles of the ischium stretch along the edge of the ischium into the clitoris legs and cover them. They form two sides of a triangle with the clitoris pearl in the upper angle. The two sides are also connected by the paired, perpendicular perineal muscles on the surface (m. transversus perinei).[2] In this way, the clitoris is connected to all of the pelvic floor (see figure 1.6 on page 16).

The average size of the nonaroused pearl or tip of the clitoris is five millimeters. This tiny area alone is home to 8,000 nerve endings that transmit sensory perceptions during sexual arousal. The surrounding area

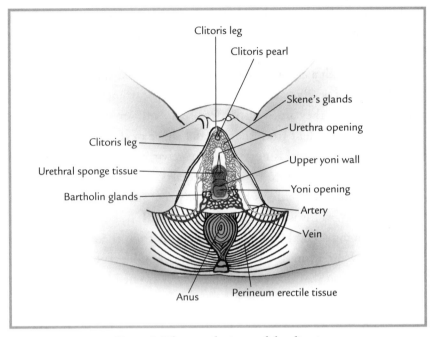

Fig. 1.5. The erectile tissue of the clitoris

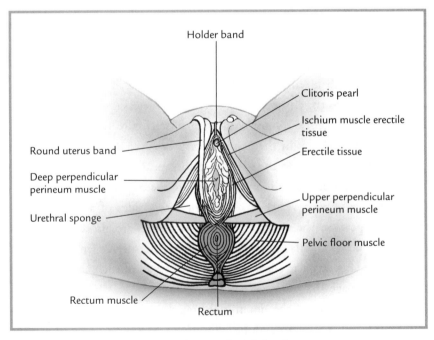

Fig. 1.6. The muscles of the clitoris

adds many more nerve endings to this number, but the female sexual center includes more than just the pearl, shaft, and legs of the clitoris. It also encompasses the inner labia, the yoni court, the highly erogenous urethra with its pronounced system of erectile tissue that can be separated only academically from the sensitive area of the upper vaginal wall, as well as the perineum, the muscles discussed above, countless nerve endings, and a web of blood vessels. This entirety has to be considered when we speak of arousal in a woman. In the sexual reaction cycle, the clitoris, inner labia, and the frontal third of the vagina form one functional unit.

When a woman is sexually aroused, her vaginal tissue fills with blood, the clitoris swells to about double its usual size, and the muscles begin to tense. When this arousal approaches its climax, the clitoris pearl stands upright and, to protect itself against too much stimulation, entirely disappears under the hood. After orgasm, the clitoris reappears.

Women usually prefer a gentle and gradual approach to the clitoris pearl. A careful touch that includes the labia often makes it easier for women to relax. Activity that is too fast or too strong can actually overstimulate the clitoris pearl and reduce its sensitivity.

Most of the women that I have massaged enjoy touch of the clitoris

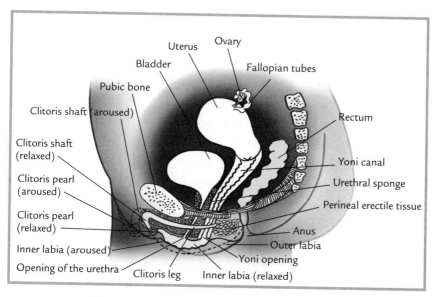

Fig. 1.7. Cross-section of the nonaroused clitoris
(and aroused clitoris—dashed line)

pearl in combination with stimulation of the G-spot, either alternating or simultaneously. During the act of making love, it is possible to gently and extensively pleasure the clitoris pearl of the partner using the tongue, while sliding one or two fingers into the yoni to stimulate the entire G-spot region.

The world *clitoris* comes from the Greek root *kleitoris,* meaning "godly" or "goddesslike."[3] I find this term extremely apt, since the clitoris is the most exciting and magical gift of nature to women, serving only to give us joy and pleasure! It has no other function. Anyone who considers this genius of nature will never be able to say that desire in women is something bad, unnatural, or unwanted. Female desire deserves to be celebrated and honored. It is the center of joy and ecstasy.

🎗 Touching the Clitoris

1. Either alone or with a partner, find a pleasant and protected room. Make sure that your or your partner's body is properly prepared, for example through a loving full-body massage (see page 108) or loving, gentle strokes.

2. You can touch your clitoris while either sitting or lying down. Find a position that is comfortable for you, and of course you can change positions while you are doing this. If you are working to touch your partner, make sure that you are in a comfortable position as well.

3. Now make gentle contact with the clitoris, first by looking at it closely and then by gently and curiously beginning to touch it. How large is the clitoris pearl, and how does it feel between your fingers? Is it more round or sharp? How does the hood feel when you touch it? How big is the body of the clitoris, and how long might it be?

4. Now use sufficient lubricant and begin to touch and stroke the clitoris gently all over. Be careful for some time, making sure to keep your touch comfortable and pleasant for your partner, even as you begin to increase your pressure slightly. If you are massaging yourself, make sure to focus on your touch, since you will probably notice that the feelings continue to change. If you are touching your partner, ask her how firmly and how fast your movements may become.

5. Every once in a while, rest your movements and remain still so that you (or your partner) can fully understand what is happening with

your feelings. What thoughts and memories are coming up? Are you feeling aroused, or rather sad and vulnerable?

6. Whatever you are feeling, allow yourself to feel it, and take deep breaths. When you close your eyes, do you see colors or is it dark? Do you feel weightless and lifted, or narrow and afraid? None of what you feel carries a specific meaning; none is particularly good or bad. The most important thing is your perception and presence. Do not judge your feelings.

7. You can now continue and think of different ways to stimulate the clitoris. For example, you can stroke up and down with your finger and thus stimulate the front of the clitoris, or you can touch it more indirectly from the side by taking the clitoris pearl between your thumb and index finger and playing with it. You can move the hood back and forth or carry out circling movements directly on the pearl. You can begin gently and increase the pressure—there are many possibilities. Play with it and see what you and your partner enjoy the most.

The G-Spot or Goddess Spot

After you have had a more intensive contact with the entire outer and visible area of the yoni, you can begin to explore the nonvisible area. As we have already noted, there is a big difference between the upper and lower vaginal walls in terms of how sensitive they are to the touch. This is linked to the fact that the upper vaginal wall is connected to the very sensitive urethral sponge. For this reason, the G-spot, which I prefer to call the Goddess spot, is not actually a specific spot, but rather an erogenous zone in the upper yoni area.

There are a number of different theories about the sensitivity of the Goddess spot. The most interesting theory claims that the nerves on the pearl run through this exact spot on their way back to the spinal cord. Regardless of theory, the Goddess spot is inside the yoni behind the pubic bone, in the area of the upper frontal wall of the yoni canal. The characteristic of the Goddess spot is that the tissue on this spot feels ribbed or hard, while the rest of the yoni wall is smooth. From the giving person's point of view, it is located toward the left side in a small indentation. In addition, there is a connection between the nerves of the Goddess spot and the bladder, which means that when this point is stimulated, a woman will often feel a (false) need to urinate.

The Goddess spot is surrounded by spongy tissue, the urethral sponge (corpus spongiosum urethrae). This tissue surrounds the urethra and serves as a protective buffer when the lingam or fingers enter the yoni. The embryonic tissue that leads to the development of the urethral sponge and associated Skene's glands in female fetuses is the same tissue that forms the prostate in males. In men, this tissue later produces prostate fluid and semen to form ejaculate.

In the case of women's sexual arousal, this tissue fills with blood, and in cases of very high arousal, a fluid can come out of the glands alongside the urethra (Skene's glands) that resembles male prostate fluid and that is referred to as female ejaculation. Female ejaculation can vary from a few drops to veritable fountains. Women who ejaculate for the first time are often afraid, as they think they are urinating. Many studies have shown, however, that this fluid is very different from urine. Female ejaculation is often described as a very joyful event, since it occurs in a moment of complete surrender when all control is relinquished.

Oftentimes, the feelings of women during the stimulation of the Goddess spot go very deep, and the resulting desire is experienced as very wide and elevating. Sexuality becomes softer and women feel themselves to be more sexually present. I personally feel my excitement much more strongly, and feel it throughout my body, when the Goddess spot is included in the stimulation. My whole being feels much more aroused.

The area of the Goddess spot, however, usually has to be found in each woman. As long as a woman is not truly in touch with this point, she will feel little or no joy from its stimulation. However, the sensations become stronger the more she learns to interact with this point. It is important to keep in mind that every woman needs time to open herself. Many women are used to a penetration of their yoni that is too fast, and unaccompanied by sufficient preparation. Some women learn to deal with this, but others may not have learned how to make sure they reach this point in time, and instead they close up further and react with pain.

The sensations on the inside of the yoni during sexual activity often depend on how receptive the woman is at that moment. Some women who complain of pain during penetration are afraid that this will have lasting negative effects on their sexuality, but when I ask them whether they experience this pain all the time, almost all of them can remember incidents of complete openness when this pain did not occur.

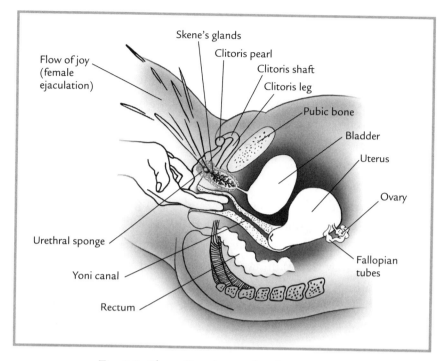

Skene's glands

Flow of joy
(female
ejaculation)

Clitoris pearl

Clitoris shaft

Clitoris leg

Pubic bone

Bladder

Uterus

Ovary

Urethral sponge

Yoni canal

Rectum

Fallopian
tubes

Fig. 1.8. Flow of joy during female ejaculation

✤ Massaging the Goddess Spot

1. Find a quiet, pleasantly warm room, and make it appealing to you and your partner with candles, relaxing music, and sensual scents.
2. Prepare your body or your partner's body for the massage. This is best done with a full-body massage (see page 108) or a sensual touching of the body followed by a massage of the outer yoni area, especially the labia.
3. To have better access to the yoni, it is best to place one or two pillows under the pelvis.
4. Use enough lubricant and place a finger on the yoni opening. Wait until the yoni opens almost by itself and it is possible to glide inside it without applying pressure.
5. When you have a finger in the yoni, use it to massage and touch the entire inner area with small circling movements, until you have lovingly touched each spot.
6. You will note that some spots are very hot. This is where unprocessed

information is stored, and you can gently release these hot spots by resting your finger on them and applying light pressure until the heat dissipates.

7. Enter into an internal dialogue and tell it to yourself or your partner. How does the stimulation of your internal yoni area feel? What emotions does it produce? Do you feel soft and vulnerable, sad, or even angry? What colors and scents do you register? Which spots do you feel particularly clearly, and which spots do you perhaps not feel at all?

8. Now search for the Goddess spot and begin gently massaging this area. Make zigzag movements and glide in and out with your finger. Feel the touch and let your breathing become deeper; allow your breath to draw the resulting energy throughout your body.

9. In the area of the Goddess spot, there can be psychological blockages. According to Taoist teachings, these are memories of faked orgasms, performance anxiety, and feelings of worthlessness. Deeper inside the vagina are anger, neediness, and memories of abortions or traumatic births. These built-up and repressed feelings can also be seen as blocked life energy, which can prevent happiness and also lead to blockages of sexual energy. Patience and loving attention in yoni massage will help to resolve these blockages.

The PC Pump

Between the yoni opening and the anus is the perineum. As discussed above, all muscles in the pelvic area play an important role in sexual arousal, since they are all connected to the clitoris. Moreover, the perineum is the starting point of a number of energy pathways, known as meridians in Chinese medicine. It is thus worthwhile to get in touch with the perineal area. A massage of the perineum increases our energy and our pleasure, especially when we also massage the area around the yoni opening.

According to Taoist teachings, the perineum is where stress and feelings of powerlessness are stored, and where they can, in turn, be resolved. Moreover, the perineal area contains a muscle that is very important for our sexual desire and energy: the pubococcygeus muscle, or PC muscle. The PC forms a muscle plate that stretches in a butterfly shape across the pelvic floor. It envelops the urethra, vagina, and anus and connects these to the ischium and legs. This muscle is best felt when we hold in the need to urinate or close our anal sphincter. Women feel it most acutely during the birthing process.

By training the PC muscle, women can significantly increase their sexual enjoyment. The conscious tensing and relaxing of this muscle, combined with conscious inhalation (during tensing) and exhalation (during relaxation), can also be used in yoni massage.

℘ Exercise for the Muscles of the Pelvic Floor

1. Sit upright and relaxed on a meditation cushion or a comfortable chair. (Do not rest your back against the chair, since you won't be able to sit properly upright in that way.)
2. Pushing your chin forward, breathe in through your mouth, and exhale through your mouth, saying "Aaahh" with your mouth wide open. In doing this, focus your attention on your pelvic floor and try to relax it. This tantric energetic breathing may give you pleasure.
3. Continue this breathing and contract your anal sphincter muscle while breathing in, relaxing it while you breathe out. Repeat this thirty times: ten times slowly, followed by ten times at a medium pace and then ten times breathing quickly. Give yourself a little time to rest and feel after this step.
4. Now, when inhaling, contract the muscles around the urethra as if you wanted to hold back your urine. Then exhale as you relax the muscles. Repeat this thirty times: ten times slowly, followed by ten times at a medium pace and then ten times breathing quickly. Again allow yourself a little time to rest.
5. Now contract your yoni opening while you are breathing in, as if you wanted to enclose a finger in it, and relax it while exhaling. Repeat this thirty times: ten times slowly, followed by ten times at a medium pace and then ten times breathing quickly.
6. Lie down on the floor, relax, and feel the warmth in your pelvic floor.

Initially, you may find it difficult to activate the different muscles independent of one another, but this is merely a matter of time and practice. Over time, you will be better able to differentiate the muscles and control them independently of one another. You can contract and relax these different muscles at any time without anyone noticing, for example while riding the bus or subway, while cooking, or while working at the computer.

The Uterus and the Uterine Cervix

The uterus is a muscular, pear-shaped organ. It is located in the lower center of the pelvis, between the bladder and the rectum. In nonpregnant women, the uterus is about three inches long. It is made up of two equal-sized parts, the uterus body and the cervix. We can establish conscious contact with the uterus in physical, energetic, and spiritual ways. The cervix extends a few centimeters into the upper vaginal canal, where you can feel it with your fingers or look at it using a speculum. Usually, women don't notice when their cervix is touched, but many report that something changes in their feelings. Most speak of a pleasant expansion or a rising internal light.

During ovulation, the cervix is at the very bottom of the vaginal canal; four or five days later it moves up again. Similarly, the structure of the cervix is different during ovulation. It is very compact at the beginning of the monthly cycle, while during ovulation it becomes softer and more permeable. With experience, one can tell by touching the cervix whether a woman is in her fertile phase. Women who use natural family planning can determine fertile days by observing the position and texture of the cervix in addition to evaluating cervical mucus and basal body temperature.

Ligaments connect the uterus to the pelvis. These ligaments are very elastic and can adjust to the changing size of the uterus during pregnancy. With its active muscle structure, the uterus also plays a role in sexuality. During sexual stimulation and orgasm, the uterus pulses with rhythmic, sexually stimulating contractions.

The uterus is the organ that clearly signals to women that we are creatures of nature and thus are bound to natural cycles. No other organ has such a profound effect on the life of a woman: The first period is the initiation to sexual maturity, which begins the transformation of girl to woman. The monthly periods reflect our continuing connection to nature, to the moon cycles, and to the rhythms of the earth. The lack of a period can signify a pregnancy, which presages comprehensive life change for women.

Pregnancy and birth are the points in life when the uterus is prob-

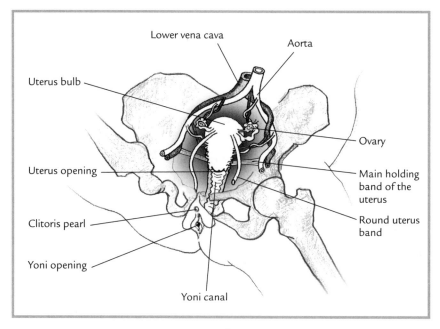

Lower vena cava

Aorta

Uterus bulb

Ovary

Uterus opening

Main holding
band of the
uterus

Clitoris pearl

Round uterus
band

Yoni opening

Yoni canal

Fig. 1.9. The uterus

ably most clearly in the consciousness of a woman. No other organ in the human body is as capable of flexibility and transformation as the uterus. Shortly before birth it can increase its size a hundredfold, yet six weeks later it can return to its original shape as if nothing had happened.

The eventual conclusion of the monthly periods initiates menopause, announcing a new and decisive part of a woman's life. This phase represents the transformation from fertile mother to wise older woman.

The shaman Maraya Haenen, who accompanied me during many stages of my own personal growth, described the processes of the moon cycle (menstruation) that takes place in our uterus as a microcosm of creation. In this way, our uterus contains within it all of the energetic information of creation. To visualize this, I think of an energetic umbilical cord that directly connects my uterus to Mother Earth. When a tree is cut down or I hear news of another capsized oil tanker polluting the sea and killing life, I can feel this pain directly in my uterus.

The uterus can be seen as an organ whose secondary function is to receive and interpret sensory information.[4] Our knowledge of the past, present, and future comes from the uterus. It is the home of our intuition and the place from which we get our "gut instincts." Women often receive information, inspiration, or creativity spurts in the form of images or dreams; these come directly from the uterus. Once a woman is truly in touch with her uterus, she is automatically linked to the entirety of creation. Native American tribes viewed a woman's "medicine dream"—a vision or dream of the future—as holy information.

The uterus is located in the abdomen, which we can think of as a type of drum. If the drum has too little tension, both energy and sound evaporate when we strike it. When a drum has too much tension, the sound bounces off without proper resonance and tone. But if a drum has an optimal tension, it can produce a strong and healing sound. If we drum for an hour or longer, we can completely enter another world, cross time, and access both the future and the past.

It is the same with our abdomen and uterus. When the abdomen is too flaccid, it cannot contain our life energy, which then dissipates. If it is too hard and tense, we are not open or receptive enough for fresh energy and new information—these simply bounce off us, like a ball against a wall. However, if our abdomen has the right tension, we can receive, contain, and process creative and inspiring energies. If we want to bring our uterus and abdomen into the right tension, hatha yoga or another body exercise program can be very helpful.

The uterus and ovaries form something of a center, a type of heart in our lower body. Much like the heart, the uterus has a connecting function between the receiving part and the active part inside of us. This is also the view in Chinese medicine, which even describes a meridian that connects the heart and the uterus.[5]

No other organ has been the subject of as many hair-raising analyses as the uterus. The famous Greek doctor Hippocrates diagnosed women with the illness of "hysteria," *hystera* being the Greek word for the female reproductive organ. With this term he described a particular state of excitement, whose cause was to be found in a "moving" uterus. The uterus was understood to be like an animal that wandered to different organs and from there caused various symptoms. Only sexual intercourse and pregnancy would mollify this animal and cause it to return to its proper place. Galen, another important doctor of antiquity, also called for the sexual satisfaction of women to treat symptoms of hysteria. During the Middle Ages, when much of culture was influenced by Christianity, doctors advocated the removal of the uterus from a woman's body as the cure for hysteria.

While today we might smile at the beliefs of doctors from those times, the truth is that even now the uterus is not valued as much as it ought to be; this is evident in many ways, including the fact that the surgical removal of the uterus (hysterectomy) is often carried out unnecessarily. The uterus is a creative, energetic, and sexually active organ that cannot simply be removed when it is deemed to have "served" its function.

✲ Massaging the Uterus

Unfortunately, it is not possible to touch one's own cervix in a relaxed position. For this reason, it is best to ask a partner to carry out this massage. If you don't have a uterus anymore, ask your partner to touch and massage the scars in this area.

Prepare a beautiful and comfortable massage paradise with everything that you want in it, and begin with a loving full-body massage (see page 108). It is very important that the entire yoni is sufficiently "awakened" before you enter the inside of the yoni temple. Now follow these instructions for the massage-giving partner.

1. Place your warm left hand in the area of the uterus on the lower abdomen of your partner and, after sufficient preparation and the application of plenty of lubricant, insert first one and then two fingers carefully and slowly into the yoni.
2. With both fingers, glide deep inside the yoni and search for the cervix. Depending on your partner's cycle, this can be very far at the top or slightly further down. Sometimes the yoni canal may feel very convoluted.
3. With both fingers you can now lightly move the cervix. Try it.
4. With both fingers, circle the cervix, while the other hand assists from the outside. There are subtle energies here that can be released through touch. Ask your partner how she is feeling.
5. As receiving partner, can you feel your cervix being touched? If yes, what does it feel like? What emotions do you feel? What images are coming to mind? Is your perception changing? But perhaps you don't feel anything. Whatever happens, simply note it and take deep

breaths, down to your uterus. Feel how your uterus is filled with fresh oxygen, and thus with new energy.

ℬ Entering into Energetic Contact with the Uterus

I recommend doing this exercise daily, ideally for a few minutes before going to sleep. It is worth it.

1. Lie down on your bed or on a quilt on the floor and relax. Rub your hands strongly against each other so that they become hot and charged with energy. Place them on your lower abdomen, directly on top of your uterus.
2. Feel how the warmth and energy from your hands flow to your uterus and thus create a connection. Repeat this two or three times.
3. Now let your hands rest on your belly and take deep breaths down into your uterus to supply this whole area with fresh energy.
4. Feel how your abdomen rises as you inhale and descends as you exhale. Focus your thoughts on your uterus and extend your contact with it.
5. Ask your uterus how it is feeling, and what it needs from you to make this contact deeper. In doing so, be completely calm and open yourself to all thoughts, colors, and pictures that may come. Do not be disappointed if your thoughts are unclear at the beginning—you will soon see them more clearly.
6. Now you can ask your uterus other questions too, anything that is on your mind at the moment. Perhaps you will receive answers in the form of images or ideas, or perhaps the next day a friend will surprise you with a book on the topic you were considering, or the question may simply resolve itself inside you without your noticing. These answers often come in completely unexpected ways. Be open and present to make sure you can receive the messages.

The Ovaries

The fallopian tubes are located at the upper end of the uterus, one on each side. Underneath their outer edges are the ovaries. The sides of the ovaries, which can be visualized as frayed ferns, catch the egg during ovulation. The egg slides from the ovary into the fallopian tube, and from there into the uterus.

We have already been in contact with aspects of female sexuality that lie beyond reach of our physical touch. Even so, the cervix gives us the opportunity to touch and observe at least a part of the uterus; the ovaries, however, are completely outside of our reach. Without physical contact, we nonetheless have an opportunity to engage in spiritual contact with our ovaries, which can be as powerful as a thorough massage. The more we recognize that body, spirit, and soul form a unit, the more we can experience a deep contact with our ovaries that is not reliant on physical touch. Energy follows attention, which specifically means that we can use our mental presence to apply an energy massage to our ovaries.

The ovaries in women correspond to the testicles in men, and the fallopian tubes to the sperm ducts in men. However, there is no male organ that corresponds to the uterus. The Müllerian-inhibiting substance in the male fetus eliminates the fetal uterus.

On the sides of the uterus, on the left and right walls of the pelvis, are our ovaries, which are about the size of walnuts. Inside the ovaries, the egg cells mature. In contrast to men, who produce up to 12 billion semen cells from puberty onward, women do not produce new eggs, since they have an ample supply of them starting from birth.

A twenty-week-old female fetus contains about six to seven million eggs; at the time of her birth about 400,000 to 500,000 egg cells remain. This dying of the eggs, caused by an inborn cell-death program called apoptosis, continues through a woman's menopause, as a sort of natural

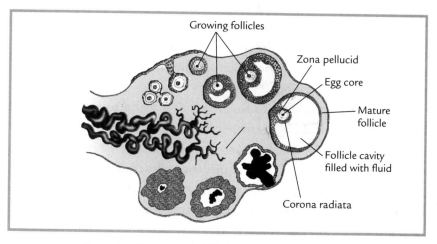

Fig. 1.10. Ovary with follicle, egg cell, and egg core

selection process. To ensure that the strongest and best eggs have enough room to grow, the lesser eggs step back and yield the field to their "sisters." In this way, about 450 eggs, the very elite, will reach ovulation. The ovaries also produce the female sex hormones—estrogen and progesterone—as well as small amounts of the male hormone testosterone. The egg itself is made up of clear cell plasma. It is the only ball-shaped cell in the entire body and looks like a sun with a shining halo. The egg cell has a magnetic effect on male sperm but does not actively move toward the sperm on its own; instead, it waits for sperm to be attracted to it. To reach the egg, the sperm has to travel a path full of obstacles and overcome a number of selection procedures. This helps to ensure that the egg will be fertilized by the best of the best.

During ejaculation, about three million sperm cells are pushed into the yoni. The cervix begins to stretch and, like a small elephant snout, dips into the seed lake and absorbs the sperm. The sperm now swim—like tadpoles against the stream of fluids—with a speed of about three to five millimeters per minute, through the uterus and into the fallopian tube. According to cell researcher Hanns Hatt, sperm cells have a sense of smell that they use for orientation on their way to the fallopian tube. The egg cells for their part give off a scent that is very similar to that of lily of the valley.[6]

If an ovulation took place in the previous forty-eight hours, the sperm in the fallopian tube encounter the egg cell after about forty-five minutes. Anatomical researchers have shown that thousands of sperm arrive at the egg at the same time and dock on the passive egg. It is thus not a race, as is often assumed, but more of a common dance, and the possibilities seem infinite. Those who reach the egg first will not necessarily be the ones to achieve the goal of fertilization: perhaps this prize is reserved for the one that seems most appealing.[7]

Apparently, the ability to finally admit a sperm to fertilize the egg is governed by a thick, light-colored membrane that surrounds the egg.[8] After careful examination, this membrane opens for a brief moment to admit a single semen cell and immediately closes up again. The other sperm no longer have a chance, and they die off. If the membrane does not find a sperm cell that meets its standards, it remains closed.

How exactly the decision is made about which is the right sperm cell is not clear. One possibility is that the soul of the future child is already present and knows which semen cell will be the best fit for the egg and for its own being, since this is the body in which the soul will be incarnated.[9] When the appropriate semen cell is admitted, both cells unite to form the fertilized egg cell—the zygote. With this union, fertilization—which many people do not know happens in the fallopian tubes—is complete.

Now it has happened, the indescribable miracle of the creation of human life. Two tiny cells, semen and egg, melt to one; two complementary halves—female and male, yin and yang, Shakti and Shiva—become one whole. Within four days this highly active cell miracle will nest in the uterus and begin its long development. Nine months later a complete, breathing, and feeling baby is born.

On an energetic level, there are important differences between the ovaries and fallopian tubes on the one hand, and the uterus on the other. The energy of the ovaries flows much faster than that of the uterus. An egg needs only fourteen days to reach ovulation, while a fetus needs nine months for its biological development.

In our ovaries, the egg cells give form to a steady ripening of new ideas that have creative potential. In this way, the ovaries represent a pinnacle of creativity that wants to be released into the world.[10] When we enter into contact with our ovaries, we can use this creativity in our lives.

According to Maraya Haenen, our egg cells—and in men, the semen cells—are the place where our unprocessed themes are stored. This "seated energy" is stored in our egg cells so that it can reach from there to the outside, for example in the next generation. Very strong themes can especially be found here, including creativity, revenge, hate, power, and powerlessness. Each form of energy will look for a way out, until it is expressed in some form.

Maraya Haenen also said that the egg cells are a place of extreme polarization, where the most negative and most positive information is stored. In this way, we are a composition of the best and worst characteristics and experiences of our ancestors.

Entering into Energetic Contact with the Ovaries

Take about five to ten minutes for this exercise every day. If you pay attention, you will surely note the effects of this exercise on the levels of creativity and joy in your daily life.

1. Make sure that you will not be interrupted, and lie down comfortably on your back on a bed or quilt on the floor.
2. Rub your hands until they are hot and charged with energy. Place them sideways on your lower abdomen above the ovaries and breathe calmly.
3. Feel how the hot energy flows to your ovaries and charges and revives them with energy. Repeat this two or three times.
4. Now rest your warm hands above your ovaries and focus your whole attention on them. The more mental presence you bring, the more intense and clear your contact will be.
5. With your mental eye, try to see your ovaries. Are they big or small, or are they different sizes? Do they feel flat or energetically charged? What color are they? Are they glowing, or rather gray and dark?
6. Ask your ovaries how they are feeling and what they would like from you. You can be sure that you will receive an answer in the form of images or a concrete feeling.
7. Begin an internal dialogue with your ovaries and feel this contact. What questions arise? Perhaps your ovaries have missed your presence.
8. Are there any memories, feelings, or thoughts that appear in this moment? What do they cause? Do they make you happy, sad, or thoughtful?

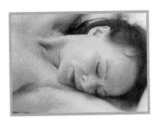

GENDER SIMILARITIES IN ANATOMY AND SEXUALITY

Surely every man has found himself wondering how it feels to a woman when, for example, her clitoris or labia are touched. Conversely, women wonder how certain touches on the lingam feel for men. Since male and female genitalia both arise from the same type of embryonic tissue, the actual differences in male and female anatomy, and in male and female sexual reactions, are far fewer than most of us assume.

It is true that the *genetic* differentiation between male and female takes place during the fusion of egg and semen cells, and during the ensuing constellation of gender chromosomes—XX for women and XY for men.[11] However, the influence of the gender chromosomes becomes apparent only in the fifth or sixth week of development, and the embryo still maintains the physical potential to differentiate into both genders. Within this first and critical phase, the development can still be artificially led in both directions, independent of genetic information.[12]

Internal reproductive organs develop from one of two duct systems within the fetus, the Wolffian and Müllerian ducts, which are controlled by genetic information in the gender chromosomes. If the embryo has female genes, the Müllerian ducts will develop into ovaries, the uterus, and the upper part of the vagina, while the Wolffian ducts will not develop. All this happens without the influence of hormones.

If the embryo has male genes, the fetal testicles produce androgens, which support the growth and development of the Wolffian ducts into the seminal vesicles, the spermatic duct, the ejaculation canal, and the epididymis. An additional hormone that causes the Müllerian ducts to recede, Müllerian-inhibiting substance, is also produced in the fetal testicles. If there is no hormonal influence on the embryo (for example through a congenital defect), the genitals will always develop as female, even if the basic genetic information is male[13] (see figures 1.11–1.13 on pages 34 and 35).

Because of this shared embryonic foundation, the sexual reactions of men and women are often similar, even if the externally visible parts of the sexual organs are very different. However, I do not agree with the commonly held view that the clitoris is the hormonal mirror of the glans penis, even though their similar appearances may lead one to that conclusion. This belief is still present in anatomy textbooks. However, the sexual reactions of the clitoris and male glans do not reflect each other. The clitoris is the most sensitive and sexually present area of most women, which cannot be said of the male glans in such concrete terms. And unlike the clitoris, the male glans has the urethra running through the middle of it, transporting urine from the bladder as well as sperm.

I find the conclusions of Sabine zur Nieden in her book *Weibliche Ejakulation* (Female ejaculation) more likely. Zur Nieden suggests that the genital eminence develops in men into the erectile tissue of the corpus

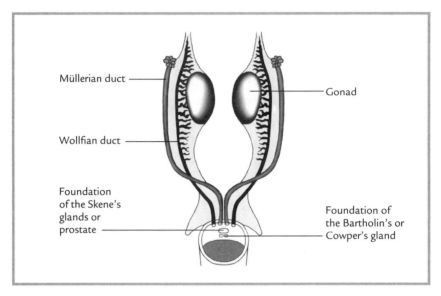

Fig. 1.11. Müllerian and Wolffian ducts: undifferentiated disposition

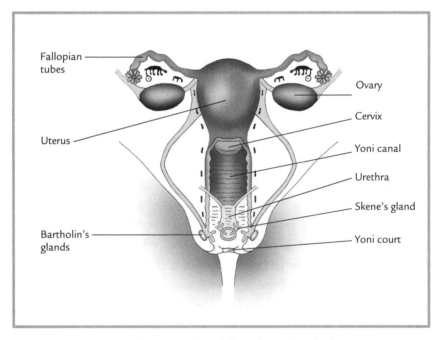

Fig. 1.12. Müllerian and Wolffian ducts: female disposition

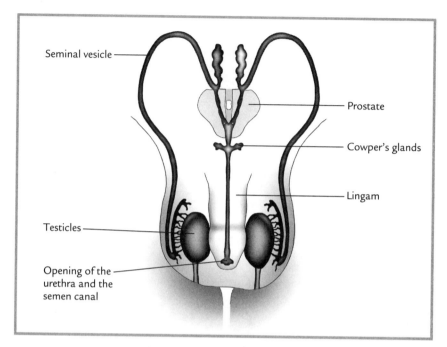

Fig. 1.13. Müllerian and Wolffian ducts: male disposition

cavernosa penis (see figures 1.14 and 1.15 on page 36), and in women into the clitoris with tip (glans clitoridis), shaft (corpus clitoridis), and legs (crura clitoridis); see figures 1.16 and 1.17 on pages 36 and 37. The "male clitoris" thus lies below the male glans (glans penis);[14] see figure 1.18 on page 37.

This also explains why the area of the frenulum is so sensitive in men. The frenulum is located on the underside of the lingam, below the spot at which the foreskin fuses with the glans. When this spot and its surrounding area are massaged well, it can be a source of great sexual stimulation for men, which mirrors the sexual sensitivity of the clitoris (see figure 1.19 on page 38).

The male glans is an inverted ending of the urethra erectile tissue (corpus spongiosum penis).[15] The corresponding female area is the entire area around the urethra (glans vulvae, female glans), which reaches into the vaginal entrance directly below the opening of the urethra.[16] This is also the area where a fluid—similar to the prostate fluid—is emitted in cases of female ejaculation. This, I believe, supports the conclusion that the male glans corresponds to the urethral sponge in women.

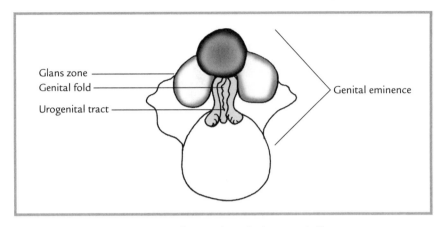

Fig. 1.14. Genitals of an embryo before sex differentiation

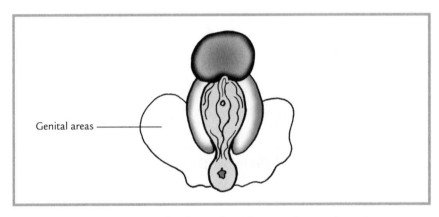

Fig. 1.15. Genitals of a male embryo in the ninth week

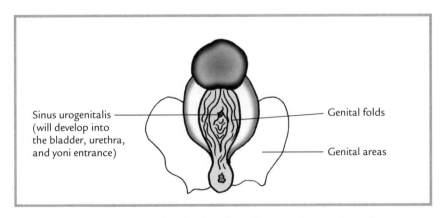

Fig. 1.16. Genitals of a female embryo in the ninth week

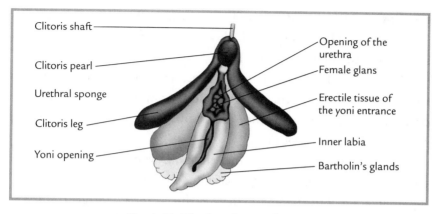

Clitoris shaft

Clitoris pearl

Urethral sponge

Clitoris leg

Yoni opening

Opening of the urethra

Female glans

Erectile tissue of the yoni entrance

Inner labia

Bartholin's glands

Fig. 1.17. The female erectile tissue

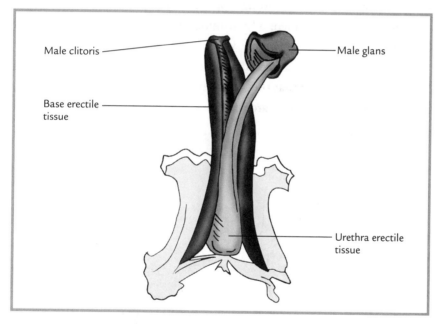

Male clitoris

Base erectile tissue

Male glans

Urethra erectile tissue

Fig. 1.18. The male erectile tissue

Based on its development, the female urethra thus corresponds to the part of the male urethra that extends through the male prostate, where a majority of the male ejaculate is formed.[17] The so-called female ejaculation originates from the Skene's glands, which are located in the urethral sponge. This intricate and highly erogenous tissue system corresponds to the prostate in men and is found in women in the upper vaginal area. It includes the Goddess spot, which we now see cannot be reduced to a single, isolated point (see figure 1.19).

The inner labia develop from the genital fold, as does the corpus spongiosum penis in men. As the genitals grow, they develop into the outer labia in girls, whereas they move down in boys and fuse with one another to form the scrotum.

It would be fair to say that the sensations women experience during stimulation of the clitoris roughly correspond to those that men feel during stimulation of the frenulum, the area directly below the glans, and the entire base erectile tissue. Men love it when the entire lingam is stimulated with an up-and-down stroke. The stimulation of the urethra region to the yoni entrance and its surroundings approximately corresponds to the stimulation of the glans in men. The stimulation of the entire Goddess spot area in the upper frontal vaginal wall in women is similar to a prostate massage in men (the prostate can also be felt and massaged via the anus). Much as women report that their orgasms are deeper, more expansive, and more intense when the area around the Goddess spot is stimulated, men

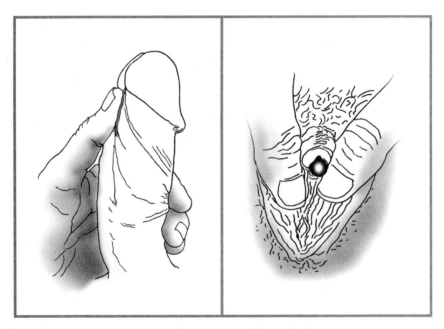

Fig. 1.19. Left: massaging the male clitoris;
right: massaging the female clitoris

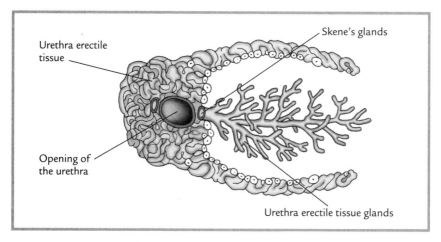

Fig. 1.20. Opening of the urethra

report that an intense prostate massage makes their orgasms last longer and makes them feel more intense—even more "female."

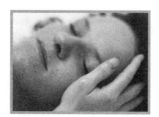

MOON TIME—THE FEMALE CYCLE

Through their cycles, women are directly tied to the strength of the moon. At the beginning of puberty, sometime between the ages of ten and thirteen, girls enter the circle of women, beginning a cyclical process that will accompany them for decades.

By making conscious contact with our menstrual cycles and their connection with other life cycles on earth, we will discover a great strength and power that resides within us. With menstruation—which I prefer to call *moon time*—we enter a new space where we can encounter our femininity. The moon time is not a physical organ but a cycle that originates in female nature. When we are conscious of this cycle, we enter deeply spiritual spaces in which we quickly recognize how our thinking becomes reality and our consciousness becomes matter. All processes of our moon time are reflected in our feelings, and thus in all projects of our life.

The menstrual cycle is directed through hormones from the brain. The part of our brain called the hypothalamus releases a chemical signal that stimulates the pituitary gland. The pituitary reacts by releasing the follicle-stimulating hormone (FSH), which then influences the ovaries. Each cycle consists of four phases:

1. The first phase, the *follicle maturing phase*, begins directly after the moon time. During this phase, FSH initiates a race among the egg follicles in the ovaries. About twenty follicles ripen simultaneously, but only one or at most two will be able to make it to ovulation; the others will give up or die off before then. As they ripen, these follicles—especially the largest among them—produce the female hormone estrogen. The follicle ripening phase, which is characterized by rising estrogen levels and low progesterone, ends with ovulation.

2. The *ovulatory phase* begins in the middle of the cycle, on about the fourteenth day, when lutenizing hormone causes the best-ripened follicle in the ovaries to break up and send its egg cell onward for fertilization. In this ovulatory process, the egg cell itself is completely passive. It is transported through the fallopian tube by means of small hairs that roll it along like a conveyor belt, in a process that takes between five and six days.

3. Now the *luteal phase* begins. During the luteal phase, the remains of the follicle left behind by the egg cell become the *luteal body*. The luteal body helps to create progesterone, another hormone. Progesterone builds the lining of the uterus, which will nourish a fertilized egg. If the egg is not fertilized, the luteal body ceases producing progesterone and eventually dies off, leading to the fourth phase of the cycle.

4. In the *menstrual phase*, estrogen and progesterone levels fall, and the uterus discards the mucous membrane, which flows out of the yoni along with blood. With this bleeding a new moon time begins and lasts for most women between three and five days.

After the moon time, the hypothalamus restarts the cycle. If an egg has not been fertilized, the period between ovulation and moon time is always about two weeks, since the luteal body, in transforming itself into a hormone-producing gland, has a limited life span of twelve to sixteen days. This means that our bleeding, independent of the duration of the complete cycle, always begins about twelve to sixteen days after ovulation.

The mucus of the cervix, produced continually by all women, clearly indicates which phase of the cycle a woman is in:

1. At the beginning of the cycle, when estrogen levels are low, there is very little mucus. It is sticky, opaque, and infertile.
2. In the middle of the cycle, estrogen levels rise and the mucus increases and becomes thinner. At the time of ovulation, when the estrogen levels are at their highest, the mucus becomes smooth and transparent—like uncooked egg white—and you will have about ten times as much of it as at the beginning of your cycle. If you pinch some mucous between your thumb and index finger, you will be able to pull it into long, shiny strings. This mucus is fertile in that it contains small vessel-like channels through which sperm can move upward. In these channels, sperm are nourished and protected until they're taken in by the uterus or excreted with the downward flow of mucus.
3. After ovulation, changes in hormone levels alter the mucus within two days. Rising progesterone and estrogen levels reduce the mucus to a thick and sticky paste, which is infertile and has a slightly yellow color.
4. During the moon time, cervical mucus flows from the yoni opening with the menstrual blood.

The Four Moon Phases and the Female Cycle

We experience the moon time physically through our blood, our excretions, and our physical reactions. In almost all romantic languages, the word for moon is female and the word for sun male. The female form represents the receptive, reflective nature of the moon. Scientists have long recognized that life on our planet would be impossible without the moon. Earth's satellite influences all waters and liquids on the planet's surface (over 70 percent of which is water), including the tides of the sea and the fluids in our bodies. The moon influences our emotions, our subconscious mind, our dreams, and our sexuality. The moon lives in our bodies, in our life rhythms, in our laps, and in our blood.

When the sun shines on the moon, the male (metaphorically) penetrates the female and makes it lively; the moon is full and light. The moon reflects this sunlight onto earth, which causes life there to pulsate and vibrate. The waters move, the seas are stormy and wild, and humans as well as animals are awake and active.

Statistically, full moon days see the most births. People become anxious and "lunatic." The living femininity in the moon's presence is difficult to grasp and thus difficult to control. Sexual energy, too, is strongest during the full moon, since this is the time when emotions flow and the soul is moved. It is the best time for going out, dancing, and making love. The full moon stimulates life. Its phase is a natural time for ovulation, for receiving life.

When no sunlight falls on the moon, it means that the male/active element does not penetrate the female/passive one, and the moon remains dark. We call this a new moon. The new moon carries within it the seeds of new life. In this time, movement on earth, in water, and in life stagnates and slows down. This is the time of retreat, the time of the subconscious, the time to process events of the past and to anticipate the future. It is also the time of bleeding, the moon time.

Between the new moon and the full moon is the waxing half moon, and between the full moon and new moon is the waning half moon. As long as no artificial interruption is made to the cycle, for example with birth control pills, many women ovulate during the full moon and have their moon time during the new moon. This cycle is called a white cycle and is considered the normal, desirable cycle. There is a strong connection with maternity and fertility.

However, our internal rhythms may change during certain times of life, so that toxins can be excreted at the best time. For some women, the best time for bleeding is the full moon, with ovulation happening during the new moon. This cycle is called a black cycle. It is linked to an internal conflict, which can be emotional and strong. Very mature women who bleed during the full moon can immediately realize their visions in this active period.

The Four Moon Phases during the Lifetime of a Woman

The entire life cycle of a woman is deeply connected to the cycles of the earth, and the four phases of the menstruation cycle are also evident in energy, feelings, and concrete experiences. The time of ovulation and the time of bleeding, along with their respective pre-phases, form a wave. This wave is mirrored in the life of a woman: from the girl phase (pre-ovulation) to the woman/mother phase (ovulation), the grandmother phase (premenstrual phase), and death (moon time).

1. **The girl** while growing up is still dependent on her parents. From them, and from the circle of women who surround her, she receives protection, nourishment, care, and inspiration. In this circle the girl playfully discovers her gifts, her talents, and her uniqueness. She learns more and more about herself and finally reaches a full awareness of her being. She knows who she is and can stand on her own in life, with confidence and conviction. This is the natural time at which a girl begins to bleed and thus enters the circle of women.

2. **The mother,** together with other women, forms a protective circle around the girls. In this phase, the things that she discovered about herself as a girl mature. Her intimacy and sexuality begin to grow in relationships with men or women. She realizes herself in accompanying and looking after her children and/or being engaged in her profession. She learns what it means to be a good mother—of creative projects, children, or other activities. The talents of the bleeding woman develop into full flower. After this time comes the harvest time, when she ceases to bleed and begins the transition to the grandmother phase.

3. **The grandmother** is mature and strong; she has become herself and now enters the collective. She is the guardian of life. A mature grandmother is free; she can move outside her circle and enter the circle of children. A mature grandmother carries an incredible beauty within her. It doesn't matter whether she has only two teeth left in her mouth, what her stomach looks like, or whether one breast sags more than the other. Her eyes and her face radiate wisdom and maturity. She carries the knowledge of life and death within her.

4. **The Kali** emerges at the time of death. The woman sheds her body and her soul enters the Kali phase. According to the teachings of Hinduism, Kali is one of the ten tantric shaktis. It is the power that controls the time of coming into and going from a physical existence. Everything comes from it and is absorbed by it. It is destruction, the godly wisdom that ends every illusion.[18]

If these phases were consciously realized and lived with celebration, life might be paradise. Unfortunately, reality is often completely different: hardly any girl receives an explanation of what menstruation is about, let alone the respect and honor that her first menstruation deserves. This topic remains embarrassing and surrounded by a lack of knowledge. Many girls hear only vague references, like "Now that you are menstruating, you can no longer play with boys, otherwise you may get pregnant." What a sad initiation into the world of women. Most women remember few days as clearly as the day of their first menstruation. Yet unfortunately this important day is often a jump into cold water, into a taboo with an endless array of unanswered questions. This is sad, but no reason to despair: we find these phases month and month again in our menstruation cycle. In this way, we always have the chance to experience the four life phases again. This applies also for women during menopause, when the cycle continues energetically. The body itself becomes our teacher—all we have to learn is how to receive our body's messages, put them into practice, and live them.

The Four Life Phases in the Monthly Cycle

1. **The girl phase:** The time when the egg grows is the most dynamic time in the cycle. This is a good time to translate ideas and projects into reality. We find it easier to deal with day-to-day life and have lots of fresh ideas. We are awake, happy, and carefree and enjoy meeting people—like a little girl at play. Our attention is focused on the outside world. Our sexuality feels new and alive. We try new things and are ready for experiments. Women who want to try yoni massage for the first time, but who are somewhat afraid of the experience, often find this open and experimental phase a perfect time to begin.

2. **The mother phase:** In this fertile phase, the egg ripens in one of our two ovaries and waits to be fertilized. Just before ovulation, some women feel a slight or strong pain in the abdomen. This is referred to as midcycle pain, and it usually goes away after ovulation. This fertile phase is our most creative time, and often the time of the cycle that women enjoy the most. Ideas and projects are looked after with care and maturity. The motherly aspect finds strong expression as we become more nurturing and look for more harmony than in our other phases. In the mother phase we are very receptive, as this is the time when the egg can be fertilized. We are easily satisfied, relaxed, and open to intimacy. Our sexual desire is at its zenith. In relation to yoni massage, this phase of the moon cycle is best for deepening our understanding of newly discovered areas of our sexuality. We find it easier to access our sexual desires, although this doesn't mean that every yoni massage during this phase will be marked by desire.

3. **The grandmother phase:** The phase from ovulation to menstruation (as long as the egg was not fertilized) is the beginning of the second half of the menstruation cycle. It ends with the onset of menstruation. The grandmother phase is an introverted time of looking back and of accessing our intuition. It is a time of intense and lively dreams. We are closely in touch with our deepest feelings, and inner truths reveal themselves in pure and unhidden ways. We are emotional during this time and convey our feelings directly. This also means that anger, tears, and aggression can surface strongly, in ways that feel out of control. However, this doesn't happen without a reason; this is the time for repressed truths to rise to the surface. Unpleasant situations, blocked energies, and unfulfilled desires demand our attention. We recognize what we truly need. We may find ourselves caught between worlds, between dreaming and waking, between internal and external, between visible and invisible things.

The much-discussed premenstrual syndrome (PMS) occurs during the grandmother phase. It occurs when we suppress or try to control our cycle. Almost 60 percent of women suffer from PMS symptoms, a figure that mirrors the imbalances and problematic relationship our society has with femininity. The premenstrual syndrome can have psychological aspects like aggression, fear, depression, irritability, and moodiness as well as physical aspects, including acne, bruises, back pain, sties, insomnia, abdominal cramps, and changes in our sex drive.[19]

These symptoms remind us that the time has come to reconcile ourselves with our femininity. If we accord enough meaning to the menstrual cycle and its different aspects, we will find that the deeper, more introverted sides of womanhood have as important a role to play as the light, extroverted, and shining sides. To become whole women, we have to recognize and deal with both sides, the light and the dark. We have to recognize the darker sides of femininity and understand them as part of our creative nature.

In this phase, sexuality goes very deep. It is strong and creative, but less playful. During this time, women should be very careful that they are saying yes to themselves and to their partner before they let themselves enter a sexual encounter. Before receiving a yoni massage, women should take care to ensure that the conditions and surroundings are pleasant, and that there is a connection of deep trust with the partner. This is a good time to allow yoni massage to bring us toward our deepest inside feelings, and even to entirely new areas of our sexuality.

4. **The Kali phase:** During the menstruation phase, the uterus expels the mucous membrane prepared for the egg, which causes our bleeding. In many cultures, this part of the cycle is called the "moon time." Now begins our most introverted and deep time of the month. This is the time to let go, in a natural way, of sadness and pain that are rooted deep in our subconscious.

The moon time in the life of a woman can be compared to the chaos described in myths before the world began to take shape. Everything is upside down, nothing can be fully controlled anymore, and from this chaos, this letting go of old weights, something new is created. However, in our over-controlled society where everyone has to function from morning to night, this is a difficult phase. Letting go and control are irreconcilable opposites. Letting go is a form of death, and death cannot be controlled. We often bury pain and sadness deep in our subconscious, causing toxins. Menstruation is a monthly cleansing process that allows women to release such toxins and griefs in a natural way.

In Native American culture, during menstruation women retreat into a moon tent—a hut that allows women to dedicate themselves fully and completely to the cleansing processes of menstruation. The idea is that Mother Earth receives this "refuse" from her daughter and composts it. In return, the daughter receives from Mother Earth fresh energy and inspiration. Macrocosmic creation, energy, and inspiration return to the uterus. Thus the microcosm of our cycle is united every month with the macrocosm of creation in a continuing process of maturation. This new inspiration from Mother Earth is transported around the body by the new blood. With each menstruation, a new piece of woman is born. Even if a woman no longer has a uterus, for example after a hysterectomy, she can energetically connect with her cycle and in this way, usually at the new moon, let go of her toxins. In some Native American cultures, there is a tradition of men entering into a sweat lodge once a month to free themselves of old weights, much as women do during menstruation.

Sexually we are very open in the Kali phase and very receptive, but also very vulnerable. Couples that have sex during this time can experience a deep feeling of connection. It is recommended, however, that you choose only partners with whom you feel safe. The menstruation phase is not a time for experiments.

Yoni massage in this phase also needs an especially intimate space, which helps to facilitate the work of letting go of deep-seated themes and blockages. The recurring theme here is letting go. Women who have problems with this—which show up, for example, in difficulties in achieving orgasm—will have easier access to the underlying themes of these problems during this phase.

The four phases described here are also mirrored in the seasons of spring, summer, fall, and winter. This shows how closely we are connected to the rhythm of nature. In the following section I show a few possibilities for women to get in closer touch with their menstrual cycle, and thus to increase the connection between their microcosm and the macrocosm of life.

⚘ Encountering Menstruation

There are different ways to become more aware of your menstrual cycle and to experience it more fully.

1. Write down the days of your cycle. Day one is the first day of your menstruation.
2. Observe the moon phases and note how they relate to your cycle. Note the moon phase when you menstruate and at the time of ovulation.
3. Observe the mucus of your cervix and note when and how it changes.
4. Every day or every other day, note the time of your cycle and how you are feeling: happy, lively, motherly, sexual, balanced—or rather withdrawn, heavy, sad, angry, uninterested in sex, tired, et cetera.
5. Observe and note whether and when you have recurring physical symptoms or pain. A woman's belly always needs protection and warmth, but especially during menstruation.
6. During the second half of your cycle, be gentle with yourself.
7. Meditate, carry out exercises, and pay attention to your dreams. During menstruation it is good to make sure you have quiet and peace. Create a pleasant place with candles, nice music, and whatever else you desire, and use it to get in touch with your uterus (see page 28). You can place your warm hands on your abdomen and take deep breaths to feel your uterus more clearly. Perhaps you will receive clear messages in the form of images or ideas. If not, perhaps this will happen in your dreams, or you will come across a message in some other way.
8. I recommend using sanitary napkins instead of tampons during menstruation, so that you can have contact with your blood. This helps to ensure that this special time doesn't pass unnoticed, or too discreetly. Of course there are situations in which tampons are very practical, but when you use them, your blood cannot flow properly.
9. If you like, find a protected place in nature where you can bleed directly into the earth. While doing this you can say a prayer or simply become very still. Here is a suggestion for a prayer. It comes from the German poet Alba Maria.

Prayer to the Great Mother

Our Mother, who is in Heaven, on Earth, and in everything,
blessed be your beauty and excess.
Bring into our hearth the key that opens the gate to love
so that we may respect the ways of all human beings.
Let the quest for forgiveness be part of our existence
so that we want to receive at this table
all those who wish to share this holy meal with us.
Let our steps lead us to higher intentions
so that the beating of our heart can become united with the
pulse of the earth.
Let us pulse in one rhythm
so that the stars may guide us during dark nights
and the sun may shine intensely on our bodies.
Hey Great Spirit.
Hey Great Mother.

The life of a woman from puberty to menopause runs in rhythms. The rhythm is determined by hormonal changes. During their twenty-eight-day cycles, women's various hormonal patterns create different mood patterns. This is one way of explaining why women have very different emotional ranges and are able to take in many emotional nuances—they live these nuances day to day in their own cycle.

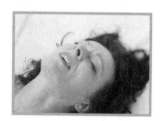

THE FEMALE ORGASM

In French, the orgasm is also called "the little death," and indeed it has something to do with dying. In the moment of orgasm you briefly give up your ego; it dies and you enter the boundary-less feeling of cosmic unity. An orgasm requires unconditional surrender; you fall into the flow of life and give up all control.

While making love with a partner or with yourself, your yoni increases in width and length and becomes wet, slippery, and receptive. The yoni opening becomes exposed, and the inner labia redden and swell. The erectile tissue of your clitoris fills with blood and your pearl slowly increases until it reaches twice its usual size.

At the same time, the uterus begins to pull into the abdomen. It also increases in size. Your nipples become erect and take on a darker color. You begin moving your pelvis forward and down, and you curl your fingers and toes. Your breathing quickens and your pulse increases. The sexual tension builds in your whole body and waits to reach its climax.

The slower and more intense the movements of lovemaking are, the more intense your feelings of desire can become. The orgasm approaches when tension and desire cause the entire string of muscles between the Venus bone (pubic bone) and coccyx to have a series of contractions. The contractions begin in the sexual area and then reverberate throughout the rest of the body. They cause an increased urge in you to reach release, which eventually prompts the orgasm. Expansion and contraction are the poles that climax in orgasm. In tantric teachings, these poles are considered similar to the beginning and end of all creation (see figure 21).[20]

Each woman carries within herself the potential for orgasm, for desire, and for limitless ecstasy. It is the birthright of each woman, of each human being, to fully and completely develop this creative and powerful potential. The climax of ecstatic desire, the orgasm is not a secret to which some women have access and others don't: it is a gift given to each woman, waiting to come to full bloom.

Let us simply decide to leave this anti-sexual era behind us and begin to give ourselves completely to this birthright of ours. Sexuality can be learned and can be healed as soon as we decide to no longer be driven by fear, or by a false code of morality that denies pleasure. Instead, we can focus our attention on ourselves—our desires, our potential, our inner truth and beauty.

Erotic fantasies are usually a very effective means of increasing sexual desire and the ability to orgasm. It doesn't matter what the specific fantasies are—the only thing that matters is that they work. Everything that works is allowed and should be used for our pleasure, as long as it doesn't impact the freedoms of others.

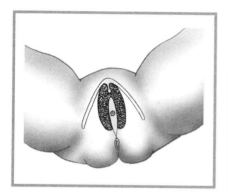

a The nonaroused clitoris

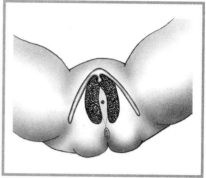

b The clitoris while being aroused

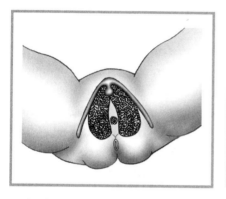

c The clitoris during the plateau phase

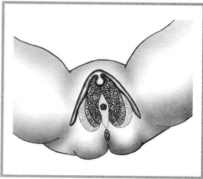

d The clitoris during the orgasm phase

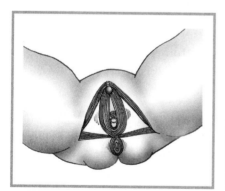

e The muscles of the clitoris during the
orgasm phase

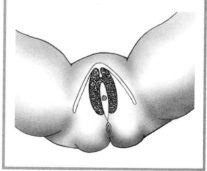

f The clitoris during the relaxation phase

Fig. 1.21. Stages of the yoni during arousal and orgasm

Many women perceive their fantasies to be dirty, perverse, or immoral and are ashamed of them. But fantasies are fantasies and have nothing to do with reality—women rarely wish that their fantasies would come true. Instead, erotic fantasies stimulate the emotions and help to increase sensations beyond their usual levels. Especially for shy or uptight women, fantasies can be a vehicle of liberation.[21]

Problems in reaching orgasm are often linked to emotional issues, like unacknowledged expectations, a need to control things, an inability to let go, or unresolved fears. These emotions can make it difficult even to recognize erotic-sexual feelings, let alone accept them. It is only when we approach ourselves with openness and without expectations that we can create a healing space. Observing what happens in reality—independent of what should happen—now becomes possible. Hidden behind this is the orgasm.

Suppressed or unprocessed injuries can cause the yoni to hurt, or to be dry and tight. These injuries can be caused by abuse, but also simply by an environment that was not conducive to a healthy sex life. Every erotic feeling will remind you of the injury, and your yoni is trying to protect you from these memories by hurting or remaining dry. This makes easy, pleasurable vaginal stimulation impossible. Your yoni is setting limits for you, which you can widen by being careful and approaching the issue with patience and trust.

To resolve such injuries you need protected and cozy spaces, as well as time and a lot of patience. Your injuries need attention to allow them to rise up from your subconscious. They want to be noted and accepted with love, so that they can then pass peacefully. Yoni massage can help to resolve these old injuries and blockages, which then creates the space for new and pleasant experiences to arise.

The level of joy we can reach during orgasm and other sexual encounters is also linked to the tension and flexibility of the pelvic muscles and to how much room you have in your pelvic floor. Muscle tension in the pelvic floor limits your sexual possibilities, while external muscle tension decreases your ability to relax.[22]

Wilhelm Reich spent a lot of time discussing the body's defenses. He referred to the way people enclose themselves in protective muscles as an armor. This body armor protects us from painful stimuli and limits our perception of emotions linked to fear. However, this protection is an illusion, since the more we protect ourselves, the more we encounter externally unpleasant situations from which we truly do need protection. This begins a vicious circle. The stronger our body armor, the less we are able to receive pleasant emotions like love, which would otherwise be received naturally and spread through the body. The consequences of this armoring are that healthy sexual responses, spontaneous joy, and sexual perception are significantly decreased. The more free and flexible your body structure, the more love, desire, and fulfillment can flow inside you. Reich called this sexual functioning potential our "orgasmic potency."

A healthy and flexible body is part of a healthy and balanced sexual life. For this, I recommend a good training of the pelvic floor, for example through a yoga class or something similar. The exercises with a yoni egg (see page 55) can also serve to significantly increase your ability to receive sexual stimuli.

Vaginal and Clitoral Orgasm

Through the many interviews that I have conducted, I know that most women prefer a combination of clitoral and vaginal stimulation. The orgasms that happen after "only" clitoral stimulation are described as explosive, sharp, exciting, and short. The orgasms that happen after "only" vaginal stimulation, in contrast, are described as soft, deep, expansive, and long. An orgasm caused by a combination of vaginal and clitoral stimulation is perceived by most women as the most intense and fulfilling kind.

In discussing vaginal and clitoral orgasms, we are still following Freud's distinctions. According to Freud, the "correct" and mature orgasm is a vaginal one, caused by the penis in the vagina. In the 1950s, the sexologist Alfred Kinsey made the assertion that the clitoris is actually the source of female desire and orgasm. He considered the vagina to be an empty space in which no nerve endings were present. It served solely as a vessel for the penis and semen.

Both points of view by themselves run deeply contrary to my experiences. I experience the female genitalia as an interconnected whole. Depending on which area I emphasize, I have different sensations.

Author Deborah Sundahl describes three kinds of orgasms in her book *Female Ejaculation and the G-Spot:* the clitoral, the combined, and the uterine orgasm. According to Sundahl, the clitoral orgasm arises from stimulation of the clitoris only, while the combined orgasm is attained by clitoral stimulation plus some penetration, or by the simultaneous stimulation of the clitoris and G-spot, or by penetration with indirect clitoral stimulation. The uterine orgasm, in contrast, is caused by deep penetration and vigorous thrusting that reaches the cervix. This form of orgasm is described as deeply satisfying and "shaking," accompanied by intense emotions.

I mostly encounter women who orgasm through a combination of clitoris and G-spot stimulation, with the clitoris often playing a central role. I think that many women still have to discover the area around the G-spot in its entirety before they can reach orgasm solely via penetration.

I often hear from women that they do not orgasm through coitus alone, even though orgasm comes easily during masturbation or manual/oral stimulation by the partner. This may be due to the fact that the clitoris pearl is located too far from the yoni entrance in many women to be stimulated during intercourse. The distance between the yoni entrance and the clitoris pearl varies among women but is usually between two and six centimeters. It is apparent that for women with a shorter distance here, it is easier to have the pearl stimulated during coitus, and therefore easier to reach orgasm than it is for women with a larger distance between the yoni entrance and the clitoris pearl.

Women who have a large distance should decide with their partner which position during coitus is best suited to stimulating the clitoris pearl, or in which position it is most comfortable to stimulate the clitoris pearl manually or with a vibrator.

However, a woman's difficulties in reaching orgasm can also have their root in a man's early ejaculation. A woman needs tender, extended foreplay in order to open herself to orgasm. If her partner ejaculates too quickly, she misses out on the opportunity to release her sexual potential. Of course there are many women who can reach orgasm as quickly—or perhaps even more quickly—than a man. But as a rule, sufficient time and sufficiently erotic foreplay are basic requirements for a woman's orgasm.

For couples dealing with issues of early ejaculation, I recommend taking part in a seminar on the topics of yoni and lingam massage, which can teach men to control and delay ejaculation. This gives both partners the opportunity to experience their sexuality in a more varied and intense way, opening the door to an entirely new quality of sexual encounter.

⅋ Exercises to Increase Desire

↻ Exercises with the Yoni Egg

Exercises with the yoni egg are used to strengthen the sexual region in order to get your sexual energy flowing freely. By improving blood circulation and muscle strength, these exercises energize your lower body. Increased circulation also makes you more resistant to infections and fungi, incontinence, and other problems of the cervix, uterus, and ovaries. As the pelvic floor is strengthened, you learn to control your muscles and become better able to use them consciously for your sexual activity. Exercises with the yoni egg thus greatly increase your potential for sexual reception and your ability to orgasm. The strengthening of your muscles will also allow you to reach a vaginal orgasm even without penetration.

As the name implies, yoni eggs are egg-shaped. They are usually made of healing stones that have positive effects on the body. They should have a hole drilled into their tip so that you can insert a small string and thus can remove the egg from your yoni at any time. The best stones for sexual exercises are rose quartz, jade, and rock crystal. Rose quartz links the first and fourth chakras and supports the development of your spiritual energies. Jade also connects the first and fourth chakras and strengthens your sexual region. Rock crystal balances all the chakras and helps alleviate muscle cramps.

Yoni eggs are available in sex shops geared toward women, in esoteric shops, and over the Internet. It is important to keep your yoni egg clean and to recharge the stone energetically at regular intervals. Before using the egg for the first time you should clean it by placing it for twenty-four hours in a glass with sea-salt water. After that, run cold water over the egg. Before using the egg, run warm water over it so that it is not cold when you insert it into your yoni. After use, it is sufficient to rinse the egg under running cold water, or to place it into vinegar water for thirty minutes. Keep the egg in a satchel or in a closed container. You can leave the egg outside during the full moon to replenish its energies.

You should not carry out exercises with a yoni egg if you are suffering from a vaginal infection or fungus or from infection in the urinary tract, or during menstruation. After menstruation it is best to wait one or two days before resuming exercises with the yoni egg. After giving birth, you should wait about six weeks so that any possible injuries have healed.

When preparing for this exercise, make sure that you will not be disturbed. If you wish, you can put on pleasant music.

1. Begin by inserting a warm egg into your yoni, with the more rounded side first. The egg can be slightly oiled if you prefer. To insert the egg, you can place one foot on a chair and bend deeply at the knees, which will facilitate insertion. Of course, it makes sense to first stimulate yourself so that your yoni has time to open.

2. With the egg inside you, sit down in a comfortable position, with your back upright and your neck straight and fully extended. Move your chin slightly down toward your chest.

3. Alternate between contracting and relaxing your love muscle (PC muscle) while counting in the following way: inhale, hold your breath, contract, and count to twelve in your head, then slowly exhale and relax. Then inhale normally and count to twelve in your head. Repeat this several times. At the beginning you should do this exercise for only a few minutes at a time, since you might otherwise end up with sore muscles.

4. After a few minutes of this exercise, feel your energy inside you. Follow the exercise with tantric energy breathing: move your mouth slightly forward, inhale deeply, and exhale with a loud and joyful *haaahhh*.

5. While continuing with this tantric breathing, contract your yoni muscles during inhalation and relax them during exhalation.

6. Repeat this exercise very slowly ten times, then ten times at medium speed, and conclude with ten times quickly.

7. Feel the effects of the exercise in your body and observe how the energy spreads throughout your whole being.

If you wish, continue with a few more pelvic exercises using the yoni egg.

1. Place your feet shoulder width apart, with your toes pointing straight ahead. Slightly bend your knees and place your hands on your hips or place one hand on the yoni and the other on the coccyx region.

2. Resume the tantric energy breathing by inhaling deeply through your

mouth and exhaling with a deep *haaahh*. Contract your PC muscle while inhaling and relax it while exhaling, just as you did in the previous exercises. Continue this breathing rhythm throughout the remainder of the exercises.

3. Begin circling your pelvis as if drawing a circle with your yoni. Circle clockwise first, then counterclockwise.

4. Now make a figure eight using your pelvis, again clockwise first, then counterclockwise.

5. Finally, lie on your back and observe energy spreading throughout your body. Allow the warmth into every part of you and let the sexual energy cause every cell to glow and rejuvenate. Say to yourself: "I am boundless energy, I am love." Then direct your energy toward your center and around the navel, using it to once again close the pelvic floor.

You can keep your egg inside your yoni for extended periods of time, if you wish. Your muscles will work with the egg, and your skin will absorb the healing effects of the stone. If you want to remove the egg, try to push it out using your yoni muscles. Pull the string only if you feel you cannot do it with your muscles alone. Perhaps you will find that you don't need the string at all.

◑ The Self-Love Ritual

The self-love ritual makes it possible for you to get to know and love your body and your yoni. You will discover your own needs, preferences, and desires and will begin a deep journey through your femininity. Only when you know your own needs and sexual preferences will you be able to identify them to your partner. This is very important in a sexual relationship, since every woman reacts differently and has different desires that her partner must know in order to be able to fulfill them.

Unfortunately, masturbation continues to be thought of as an unusual thing for women. The act is often viewed as a sign of a lack rather than as something worthy in its own right, and many people think of it as a last resort, to be employed only when there is no "other way" to release sexual tension. However, it is important to be able to enjoy and celebrate our sexuality at any time, whether in or out of a relationship, and often. Masturbation can help us to feel whole and independent with our sexual potential.

Create a pleasant, warm room in which you will not be disturbed. If you wish, decorate it with everything that gives you joy—flowers, music, beautiful objects, or anything you want. When you have enough time and peace, you can begin with the previous yoni egg exercise to prepare your pelvis for a sexual touch, and to help make your sexual experience more intense.

1. Begin by lying down naked and exploring your whole body with both hands. Gently touch your face, your ears, and your lips. Slide your hands down and rest them on your throat and shoulders. Caress your breasts in the way you like, sometimes gentle, sometimes strong. Play with your nipples; do anything you like.

2. Continue on and caress your belly. Sit up a little and stroke your legs, your feet, and your toes on both sides of your body.

3. Now approach your yoni by playing gently with your Venus hairs and by touching the outside of your yoni. Place both hands on your yoni and press them rhythmically, thus gently stimulating the clitoris. Gently rub lubricant on your clitoris, and carefully and gently massage first the outer and then the inner labia. Also include your pelvic floor, your perineum, and your anus in this massage. This is easier if you put down your feet and slightly raise your pelvis. You can place a pillow under your pelvis to make it easier for you to touch yourself all over.

4. Now touch and gently stimulate the clitoris in whichever way is pleasant for you. Begin slowly and with a light, playful touch. Follow the rising excitement, noting the pulsing in your body and the quickening of your pulse and breathing. If you would like, you can now also use a dildo or a vibrator.

5. Give yourself plenty of time, not only focusing on your orgasm, but trying also to fully understand the course of your arousal and maintaining it for as long as possible. Don't put pressure on yourself and don't be disappointed if you feel only a little aroused. Simply note what you feel, what is possible, and build on this experience.

6. Now begin to circulate your sexual energy in the Microcosmic Orbit (see page 84), using both your imagination and your breathing. Visualize your energy flowing up the spine as you inhale, and down the front of your body to your yoni as you exhale. Tense and relax the PC muscle (love muscle) several times as you do this.

7. Play with your arousal curve, letting the energy rise as far as possible until just before orgasm, and then distributing it through deep breathing, with both hands, and with the power of your imagination, throughout your whole body. Repeat this several times.

8. If you would like and can do it without tension or effort, you can now reward yourself with an orgasm, distributing this strong energy and allowing it to flow throughout your body. Perhaps you would like to begin anew and to experience several orgasms one after another.

9. Another option is to consciously not orgasm, but instead to carry out an energy exercise at the height of your arousal called the Big Draw (see page 85). This is an especially pleasant option for women who are not reaching orgasm yet. You can also carry out the Big Draw after orgasm to distribute energy throughout your body.

2

Energetic and Spiritual Basics

My hands

Touched in my depth
Flow through the evening I
Into the night
The moon in silver
Pulls me from my dream.

Breathing
Breathing feels like waves
On my shores
Flowing through the breathing night
Flowing through your nearness
Letting my hands do their duty
To respond
To the question of your body
Through the waves
Into the depths

And it does not stop
And it does not stop.

— ANTONIA ALARIS

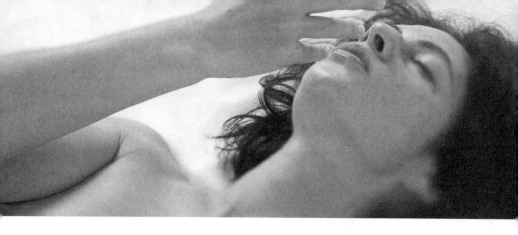

YIN
AND YANG

Many people limit their sexuality to the physical realm. However, we have the opportunity to deepen and refine this experience by consciously directing our energy. In the following chapters about yin and yang, the chakras, and breathing, I want to invite you to discover and use—through better understanding and practical exercises—the infinite energetic potential that rests in each of us.

To more consciously use our powerful sexual energies for our personal growth, our health, and our joy in life, it helps to familiarize ourselves with the ancient Chinese knowledge of yin and yang. In our bodies and in our thoughts, feelings, and actions, there are two contrasting yet complementary forces; they always appear together and they create a dual structure for all things in the universe. In Taoism, these polar forces are called yin and yang, and the balance between them is called Tao. The Tao symbol illustrates how these forces interact: The dark part symbolizes the yin, the light part the yang. The wave that separates the two shows that yin and yang flow into one another, while the small points show that one is rooted in the other. Yin nourishes yang, yang protects yin. Yin and yang always exist next to each other and flow into each other.

At certain times in our life, we will need more yang qualities such as clarity, activity, and goal orientation, while other times call for yin qualities such as connection, wholeness, intuition, and calm. The more we are able to bring these two poles into a flowing rhythm, the more balanced and harmonious our way through life will be.

Yin	Yang
Woman	Man
Receiving principle	Giving principle
Moon	Sun
Earth	Sky (air)
Water	Fire
Night	Day
Moisture	Dryness
Inside of body	Outside of body
Exhaling	Inhaling
Subconscious	Conscious
Calm	Activity
Cold	Warmth
Contracting principle	Expanding principle
Taking in nourishment	Excretion
Attraction	Repulsion
Feeling	Thinking
Material	Spiritual
Softness	Aggression
Quiet	Loud
Physical: underfunctioning	Physical: overfunctioning
Death	Life

Each breath of energy consists of both yin and yang, of male and female, of minus and plus. It is the same with our body, which consists in equal parts of yin and yang energies. What we see in figure 2.1 (opposite) is yang. It is the outside and protects the yin. That is why in situations of danger we often instinctively show our backs—our outside—and protect the front, our yin side. Everything that is covered, not visible, and protected in the illustration is yin. Yin is inside and nourishes yang.

The front of our body is thus yin, and the back yang. Our right side

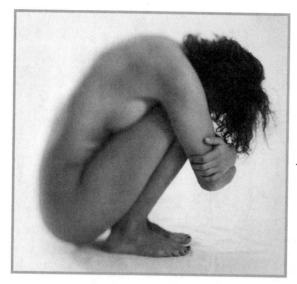

Fig. 2.1. Body in the fetal position

(which is controlled by the analytic-rational left part of our brain) reflects yang, while our left side (controlled by the holistic-intuitive right side of our brain) is yin. Our upper half, roughly from the navel upward, faces up toward the sky and thus corresponds to yang, while our bottom half, rooted in Mother Earth, is yin. Thus, the right, upper, and back parts of our body have the strongest yang qualities, while the left, lower, and frontal parts of our body have the strongest yin qualities (see figures 2.2 and 2.3 on page 64).

The yin energy (front and inside) flows upward, while the yang energy (back and outside) flows downward. We have different ways to consciously harmonize the strengths of yin and yang in our bodies and in our minds. We very directly experience their flowing rhythm during a massage that follows the flow of energy in the body. This means that we stroke the front and inside parts of our body, such as the insides of our arms and legs, upward, while we stroke the back of our body and the outer body parts such as the outsides of our legs and arms downward. You will quickly notice the resulting balancing of energies in the body, which will help you feel relaxed and protected (yin), as well as strong and vivacious (yang).

Following the flow of energy is especially effective in this massage when it is combined with deep and conscious breathing, which allows us to be more aware of the feelings, emotions, and thoughts that arise during the course of the massage. These experiences can then be integrated into

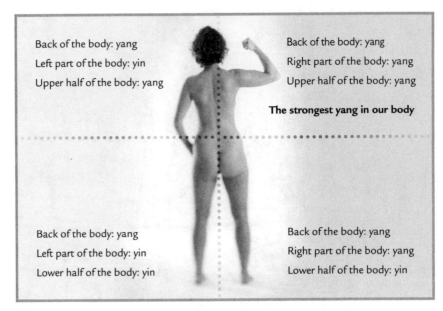

Back of the body: yang
Left part of the body: yin
Upper half of the body: yang

Back of the body: yang
Right part of the body: yang
Upper half of the body: yang

The strongest yang in our body

Back of the body: yang
Left part of the body: yin
Lower half of the body: yin

Back of the body: yang
Right part of the body: yang
Lower half of the body: yin

Fig. 2.2. Yin and yang in the body: on the back

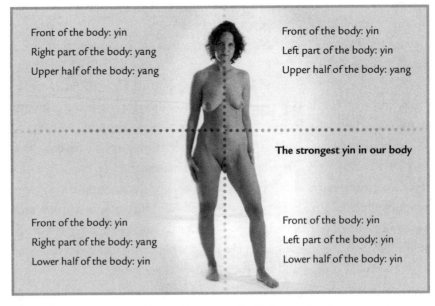

Front of the body: yin
Right part of the body: yang
Upper half of the body: yang

Front of the body: yin
Left part of the body: yin
Upper half of the body: yang

The strongest yin in our body

Front of the body: yin
Right part of the body: yang
Lower half of the body: yin

Front of the body: yin
Left part of the body: yin
Lower half of the body: yin

Fig. 2.3. Yin and yang in the body: on the front

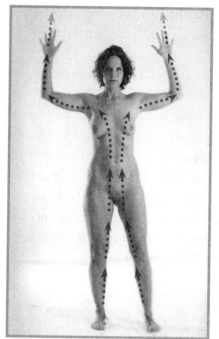
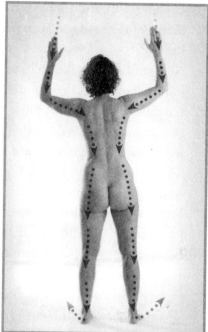

Fig. 2.4. Circulation of yin energies in the body

Fig. 2.5. Circulation of yang energies in the body

our sexuality, allowing us to experience a depth, intensity, and clarity that we might not otherwise have thought possible.

℘ Becoming Conscious of the Energy Cycle in the Body

Ask your partner to do the following exercise with you. The exercise aims to help both of you become aware of the cycle of energy and also prepares you for learning the full-body massage and honoring ritual that begins every yoni massage (see page 100).

1. Stand behind your partner, and with your hands flat, stroke down her back (but not on the spine itself) and down the back and outsides of the legs to the feet.
2. Stroke the feet and use your hands to glide from the insides of the feet up along the insides of the legs, then across the stomach and between the breasts.

3. Use both hands to continue stroking through the armpits, down the insides of the arms and across the palms, and then down to the fingertips.

4. Now stroke across the backs of the hands and arms, from the fingers to the elbows, and then up to the shoulders.

5. Carefully glide from the throat across the face and over the back of the head, then once again down the back until you return to the outside of the legs by the feet. Begin anew and repeat the entire sequence three times.

6. To conclude, gently press against your partner from behind, and place your right hand on her lower abdomen and your left hand on her heart. Make sure that you have a firm stance so that your partner can lean against you without falling. Breathe with your partner, adopting her rhythm to deepen the breaths. This moment creates a strong feeling of connection and safety.

To further harmonize the yin and yang during a massage, and especially a yoni massage, you can also breathe along the Microcosmic Orbit, a technique that is explained later in this chapter (see page 84). Also called the Small Energy Cycle, the Microcosmic Orbit is the main energy channel in our bodies. It is called microcosmic because it is considered a microcosmic reflection of macrocosmic processes like the tides. Just as an electrical main supplies all the lines that branch from it, the Microcosmic Orbit in our bodies supplies all the energy pathways that the Chinese call meridians.

The cycle consists of a back channel, called the Governor Vessel, and a front channel, called the Conception Vessel. The Governor Vessel supplies the yang meridians and runs from the tip of the coccyx up along the spine and neck to the top of the head, then down along the midline of the face to the gums. The Conception Vessel supplies all the yin meridians. It runs along the front of the body from the tip of the tongue, over the throat, and down to the pubic bone and ends at the perineum. The Microcosmic Orbit is closed by pressing the tongue against the soft palate to form a continuous energy loop.[1]

The yang energy of the Governor Vessel flows upward and the yin energy of the Conception Vessel runs downward. Thus, the energy in the Microcosmic Orbit flows differently than it does in the rest of the body, where yang energy flows down and yin energy flows up.

Our sexual life is one place where we experience the two strengths of yin and yang quite clearly. We approach orgasm when the two poles of tension (yang) and relaxation (yin) reach their climax and push us toward a resolution (orgasm) that melts the two poles into each other. For this reason, lovemaking can be more stimulating and erotic when we understand how to glide from giving activity (yang) to receiving pleasure (yin). We love to seduce and to be seduced, just as we love it when a partner gives him- or herself over to us entirely and opens with trust. When we can move from being the giver to being the receiver and allow ourselves to be pleasured until every last doubt and tension leaves our body, we will feel fulfilled and nourished on all levels.

Of course it is also possible to divide the two poles in a relationship, with one person taking over the receiving part and the other the giving part. To feel happy, these two people will then always need each other, which can lead

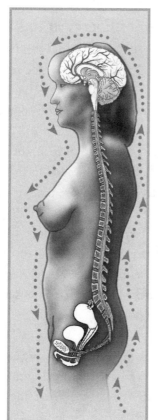

Fig. 2.6. The Microcosmic Orbit

to a dependency. We will experience our lives and our sexuality more intensely and with more confidence if we allow both these poles to melt within ourselves. In this way, we are independent in all ways, including in our sexuality. We experience the full breadth of our emotions and are more flexible and balanced in our actions. The polarity of yin and yang is also reflected in the structure of the yoni. According to this view, the clitoris represents the yang principle, which is why an orgasm that is predominantly rooted in the clitoris can also be called a "male" orgasm. It is an explosion: short, strong, and sharp. Our vaginal canal, including the Goddess spot and the urethral sponge, represents the yin principle, which is why a vaginal orgasm is a "female" orgasm: it is expansive, rolling, deep, and long. No wonder that a combination of clitoral and vaginal stimulation is considered by most women to be the deepest, most holistic, and most fulfilling orgasm of all. To become aware of this difference, I recommend that women practice both types of stimulation, initially one after the other, then combining the two.

ॐ Becoming Aware of the Flow of Energy in the Yoni

1. Begin by stimulating your clitoris. You will find a number of ways to do this described on page 18. Pay attention to the sensations this causes.

2. Now spend some time with stimulating your Goddess spot, as described on page 21. It may make sense to use a dildo for this. You may need some practice before you can really enjoy stimulation of your G-spot; it usually needs to be awakened before it can reveal its joyful pleasures. Again, note the sensations you feel and compare them to how you felt when you stimulated your clitoris.

3. Conclude by combining the two forms of stimulation, using one hand to stimulate your G-spot and the other to stimulate your clitoris. What do you feel when the two sensations combine inside you? Take enough time to feel the aftershocks of these sensations and note any thoughts or feelings that you might have.

Oftentimes, problems with our sexuality or with orgasm are rooted in an imbalance of yin and yang. If we have too much yin and too little yang, we lack arousal. Though we are wonderfully soft and open, a lack of yang energy can render us unable to build up the inner tension that is necessary for arousal. On the other hand, too much yang and too little yin may leave us unwilling to give of ourselves. We cannot let go and are thus unable to find release despite our high arousal. Some women can experience both of these extremes during the course of a single yoni massage.

I recently gave a yoni massage to a woman who had great difficulty becoming aroused. After some trying and intensive breathing, she then managed to reach arousal. But due to a fear of losing control, she was unable to let go of the tension she had built up and couldn't relax, which in the end prevented her from reaching orgasm.

These extremes can be brought to balance as we become more aware of the cycle of energies within us. If we make a decision to favor constructive thought and new experiences, we can let go of old structures and patterns and risk something entirely new, healing, and powerful. Massages, breathing exercises, curiosity, and a willingness to experiment greatly support this process.

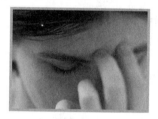

THE CHAKRAS

In the preceding section, we acquainted ourselves with the ancient knowledge of yin and yang to help harmonize the flow of energy in our bodies. Now we turn our attention to work with consciousness. How can we use our sexual energy to strengthen our mental presence and expand our consciousness?

This was also the central question that faced spiritual searchers in India thousands of years ago. In response, they developed valuable teachings about the chakra system. The word *chakra* comes from Sanskrit and means "wheel" or "circle." The chakras are roughly circular centers of energy and consciousness in the human body. According to some sources there are a great many of these energy centers in our bodies, but I will limit the following section to a discussion of the seven main chakras that share the path of the Microcosmic Orbit, which we described in the previous section.

The chakras are fine-substance energy fields that cannot be touched but can be seen by some people. Each chakra is linked to one of the following hormonal glands: pituitary gland, pineal gland, thyroid gland, thymus gland, adrenal gland, pancreas, and genital glands (ovaries or testicles). Both functionally and energetically, the chakras influence all levels of our existence: our consciousness, our emotions and thoughts, as well as the physiological processes in the body and our flow of energy. Chakras also have a significant influence on how we experience our sexuality.

We all know the different feelings and states of consciousness that we can experience during sex. According to chakra teachings, these states of consciousness change depending on which chakra is most energetically and spiritually present. Our sexual experience and behavior become more sophisticated as we learn to shift our focus from the lower chakras to the higher ones.

1. In the first chakra we experience a deep desire to use our sexual energy to achieve release. This kind of desire is wild and animalistic, and it tends to drive our actions.

2. In the second chakra we use our sexual energy in more creative and conscious ways. We are strong and filled with desire.

3. In the third chakra, we have a more subtle way of experiencing our sexual energy. We recognize it as personal charisma, self-expression, and self-confidence. We are capable of controlling our emotions in love and of participating in relationships that are based on equality.

4. In the fourth chakra, which is related to the heart, we experience the wish to become one with our partner.

5. In the fifth chakra we know what we want and can express our needs in spiritual, physical, and sexual ways.

6. In the sixth chakra, we experience sexuality in a very pure and deep way. We are clear with the other and connected to him or her in a feeling of freedom and space.

7. In the seventh chakra we are able to celebrate a truly cosmic union on all levels.

The main energy canal that runs along the spine and is known to Taoists as the Microcosmic Orbit is called Sushumna by the yogis. The Sushumna canal runs from the base of the spine—the coccyx—all the way to the top of

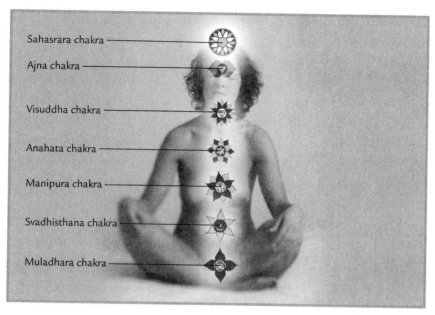

Sahasrara chakra

Ajna chakra

Visuddha chakra

Anahata chakra

Manipura chakra

Svadhisthana chakra

Muladhara chakra

Fig. 2.7. The chakras

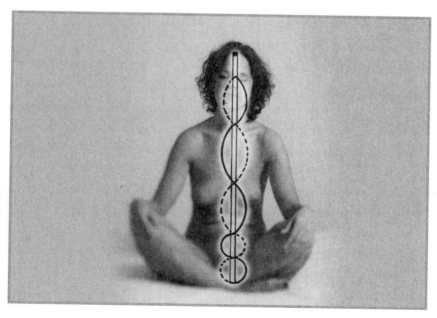

Fig. 2.8. Sushumna, Ida, and Pingala

the head. In this canal, our sexual energy flows upward, passing through all of the chakras and back down along the midline of the front of the body.

On both sides of this canal are two further energy canals, or *nadis*, which in tantric philosophy are called Ida and Pingala. Ida represents the "negatively" charged moon energy, which reflects the female aspect. Pingala is the "positively" charged sun energy, which represents the male aspect. From an observer's point of view, the Ida originates on the right side of the base of the spine, while the Pingala originates on the left side. Like snakes, these two energy canals continue upward, circling along the Sushumna and crossing it at the important points of the chakras.

Consciousness, development, and growth are encouraged when we activate these energy centers and bring the dual strengths of Ida and Pingala into unity with one another. Conscious, tantric sexuality means deepening our pleasure, experiencing it more intensely and for longer periods of time. This we can achieve when we refine our sexual energy by letting it flow up along the spine and through the chakras. An exercise to help this is described below. In addition, every yoni massage activates the chakras with conscious breathing, thereby offering real opportunities for growth and expanded consciousness.

ℰ Cleaning and Energetically Stimulating the Chakras

With this exercise we attain spiritual clarity and energy. If you choose, you can begin each chakra session with the alternate-nostril breathing exercise described on pages 80–81. This breathing exercise stimulates all chakras and cleanses the nadis, Ida and Pingala.

1. Lie down on your back and close your eyes. Feel yourself being carried by the earth and let your body come closer to the ground.
2. Inhale through the nose and exhale through the mouth while visualizing your healing warmth flowing into the chakras with each breath you exhale. Concentrate on this flow of energy.
3. Place your hands on your groin (first chakra). With a conscious and deep inhalation, take in the cosmic life energy (prana), and let it flow into the first chakra as you exhale. Visualize a warm red stream of light. Continue this for five to seven deep breaths, remembering

to inhale through the nose and exhale through the mouth.

4. Now place your hands on the area below your navel (second chakra). With a conscious and deep inhalation, take in the life energy, and as you exhale, let it flow to the second chakra. Visualize a warm orange flow of light. Repeat for five to seven deep breaths.

5. Place your hands on the solar plexus area above your navel (third chakra). With a conscious and deep inhalation, take in the life energy, and as you exhale direct it toward your third chakra. Visualize a shining yellow ray of energy. Repeat for five to seven deep breaths.

6. Now place your hands on your chest at the level of your heart (fourth chakra). With a conscious and deep inhalation, take in the life energy, and with your exhalation direct it toward your fourth chakra. Visualize a smoky green stream of light. Repeat for five to seven deep breaths.

7. Now place one hand on top of the other on your throat (fifth chakra). With a conscious and deep inhalation, take in the life energy, and let it flow to the fifth chakra as you exhale. Visualize a light blue stream of light. Repeat for five to seven deep breaths.

8. Place the middle finger of each hand on the third eye between the eyebrows (sixth chakra). With a deep and conscious inhalation, take in the life energy, and let it flow through your fingers into your third eye as you exhale. While doing this, visualize a dark blue stream of light. Repeat for five to seven deep breaths.

9. With your left palm, touch the highest point of your head (seventh chakra) and place your right hand over your left. With a deep and conscious inhalation, take in the life energy, and let it flow into your crown chakra as you exhale. While doing this, visualize a white stream of light. Repeat for five to seven deep breaths.

10. Now place both hands on the ground next to your body and take about five minutes to feel the aftereffects of this exercise.

11. Sit upright with your legs crossed on a meditation cushion and hold your ankles. Now you will connect all your chakras with one another through conscious breathing.

12. With a deep and conscious inhalation, visualize your breath traveling upward from your coccyx along the spine.

13. Then visualize your breath flowing downward from the top of your head along the front of your body to your coccyx as you exhale.

14. Allow a flowing breathing cycle to be established that supplies your entire being with fresh energy.
15. To conclude, lie back down on the floor and feel the energy flow through your body.

When we cleanse and harmonize our chakras through conscious use of our sexuality, we create tangible effects on our behavior and on the way we view and deal with events in our lives. Each of us has a primary connection with a specific chakra, which corresponds to the level of consciousness with which we view the world. Our being responds to this point, and we feel at home here. We continue to resonate with this particular chakra until everything at this level of consciousness is understood, explored, and internalized. Then we can proceed to the next level.

In contrast, our daily emotions, experiences, thoughts, and impulses can originate from any of the chakras and can switch from one chakra to the next. Our experiences are interpreted, however, from the perspective of our primary state of consciousness.

Each chakra is linked to an element. For example, the first chakra corresponds to earth, the second to water, the third to fire, the fourth to air, and the fifth to ether. Energies in the sixth and seventh chakras are so subtle that they are no longer influenced by any element. In each chakra, our consciousness, thinking, and behavior are marked by the qualities of the corresponding element; we become increasingly refined as we move from one level to the next.

1. **Earth** gives us the ground on which we stand, and on which we build our houses. Earth nourishes us and gives us a base from which to act. If our consciousness is in the first chakra, we tend to interpret our experiences based on the needs of survival. We deal with the material level of living.
2. **Water** keeps us alive, cleanses us, and gets our feelings flowing. If our consciousness is in the second chakra, we interpret our experiences through the lens of our bodies and our vitality. We deal with the sexual and physical levels of living.
3. **Fire** warms us and heats our emotions. If our consciousness is in the third chakra, we interpret our experiences from an ego-

focused perspective; we feel strong emotions and identify strongly with societal norms. We deal with the individual level of living.

4. **Air** gives us the breath of life and helps us process our experiences. Air connects all beings to the earth. If our consciousness is in the fourth chakra, we emphasize empathy, love, and self-expression in our experiences. We deal with a connected way of living.

5. **Ether** is the highest element and the symbol for space and expansiveness. In the fifth chakra, communication, self-expression, and identity are important characteristics of our experiences. It is a communicative level of living.

6. On the level of the sixth chakra we interpret our experiences in connection with our mental abilities and elevated self-consciousness. It is a spiritual way of living.

7. On the seventh charka we are connected with the experience of self-fulfillment or enlightenment. It is a collective way of living.

We can see how the primary chakras inform our lives in the following example: Imagine that Person A is "at home" in the heart chakra (fourth chakra) and Person B is "at home" in the earth chakra (first chakra). Now imagine that both people have an experience based on the fire chakra (third chakra). Both are in a situation of heated emotions, of power and powerlessness, and of societal identification. Person A will attempt to solve the problem based on a feeling of connected togetherness, while Person B will act on clear needs of survival, emphasizing material security and life or death choices (in either the tangible or the metaphorical sense).

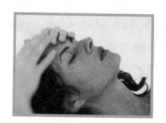

BREATHING AND CONSCIOUSNESS

To breathe is to live; deep breathing can also help consciousness and cleansing. Appropriate breathing can help to distribute the energy that builds up during a yoni massage, thereby increasing our consciousness, facilitating inner cleansing, and generating energy. We can positively influence the transformation of our sexual energy with our imagination and certain exercises.

Conscious breathing allows us to experience life as it happens, moment to moment. Our body and our consciousness melt together to form a unified whole. The rhythm and depth of the breath stand in close relation to our physical, emotional, and spiritual health. When we pay attention to breathing as a process, we will quickly note that it occupies a place somewhere between our conscious and subconscious awareness and thus forms a bridge between these two parts of our being. This middle space makes breathing an ideal arena for studying the practical and experience-oriented part of consciousness.

Breathing is subconsciously regulated by the brain stem. Although we can consciously influence our breath by increasing or decreasing respiration, the multilayered sequence and coordination of events that regular breathing requires would be impossible to accomplish consciously. Breathing also influences the heart rate. When we hold our breath for an extended period of time, our heart rate lowers, giving the heart muscle a longer rest period.

Deep and conscious breathing causes an activation of the nervous system—just as sexual touch does. To some extent, the respiratory and sexual arousal systems work together. Yet it is more difficult to focus erotic energy than it is to focus the breath. When we hold our breath, our erotic energy continues to flow, spreading throughout our bodies and emanating from within to the outside. On the other hand, we can use our breath to soften our erotic energy and make it flow, allowing us to steer it more consciously. Just as an oven creates heat in a house, the yoni creates heat in our bodies. In this sense, our breathing can be compared to the heating system that distributes the heat throughout the house, circulating arousal throughout the entire body.[2]

If a woman does not pay attention to her breathing when she is touched, then her attention will wander where it always has. For example, if a young person feels guilty while masturbating, her attention is absorbed by thoughts of shame, which impedes the free flow of sexual energy. Conscious breathing thus offers a chance to change typical sexual behavior and thought patterns and to focus attention solely on sensations and the body's own messages.[3]

By breathing consciously, we enter new spaces of perception. We are able to look at our behavior patterns, blockages, problems, and thought patterns from a different perspective—from another level of consciousness—which changes their energy and allows us to envision ways of resolving them. Certain problems cannot be solved by running away; the more we try to leave these difficulties behind, the more destructive their effects will become in our lives. Instead, we can learn to look at them from a different perspective. This will change their energy, and the problems will go away by themselves.

In the following section I describe a few breathing exercises that can be used before or during a yoni massage. Before you begin with these exercises, however, it is useful to give some thought to the sequence of healthy breathing. The breathing cycle consists of three parts: inhalation, exhalation, and the pause between the two. Inhalation is the active expansion of the chest, which fills the lungs with fresh air. Exhalation is (usually) the relaxation of the chest muscles, which causes the lungs to empty.

The first station that a breath passes on its way into our body is the nose. Contact with the mucous membranes inside the nose warms inhaled air to body temperature and enriches its humidity. The fine hairs in the nose filter foreign matter such as germs and dust from the air, preventing them from entering more deeply into our bodies. The primary breathing principle should thus be to breathe through our noses.

Other principles of healthy breathing include the following:

- The back should be straight.
- The shoulders should be relaxed.
- The face, jaw, and tongue should be relaxed.
- Inhale fully and deeply, causing your internal space to expand.
- The pelvis should open during inhalation.

There are four types of breathing:

1. **Deep pelvic breathing** activates the lower parts of our lungs especially, less so the middle and upper parts.

2. **Chest breathing** activates only the middle parts of our lungs.
3. **Upper chest or collarbone breathing** activates only the upper parts of our lungs.
4. **Combined breathing** uses the full range of the lungs. This is the ideal type of breathing.

ℬ *Preparatory Breathing Exercises*

☙ Deep Pelvic Breathing

Fundamentally, deep pelvic breathing is our most natural breath. We breathe this way when we are not disrupted by external influences of any kind. This type of natural breathing can be beautifully observed among infants and also in cats, who often stretch out on the floor and regenerate their energies using pelvic breathing. A breath can indeed reach all the way down to the pelvis.

Yoga emphasizes the importance of exhalation. Only those who exhale fully can inhale properly. However, exhaling completely does not mean using the abdominal muscles to press out every last bit of air from our lungs. Conscious exhalation is done by slightly opening our mouths and saying *ha-ha-ha*, almost inaudibly, in short intervals. Exhaling in this way calms the heart and our breathing organs. It promotes concentration and calm, deep relaxation, thus leading to increased energy.

Deep pelvic breathing is a very intense process and a great joy. By practicing it, you will have a new appreciation for your pelvic region. Pelvic breathing means bringing consciousness, sensuality, receptiveness, and feelings all the way down to your yoni. This type of breathing automatically helps you to work on resolving blockages in the pelvic region.

1. Lie down comfortably on your back. Move your head and feet gently back and forth to make sure that you are truly relaxed. Place one hand on your yoni—ideally in such a way that you can also feel the perineum—and one hand on your stomach.
2. If you like, you can bend your knees slightly so that your feet are flat on the floor, about hip-width apart. This prevents an arched back and facilitates deep pelvic breathing.
3. Close your eyes and begin with the *ha-ha-ha* exhalation described above.

This causes the abdomen to fall and become ready for inhalation.

4. Now begin inhaling slowly and steadily through your nose. Feel how your breath coolly touches the back of your nose and moves through your throat. This sensitive inhalation through the nose allows us to breathe more and more deeply into our pelvic area. Follow this inhalation with undivided attention down to the perineum. In this way you will fill your entire pelvis. Your belly will fill like a balloon with fresh oxygen, and your abdomen will rise.

5. Now exhale slowly through your nose. Your abdomen will fall and you can begin the next round, beginning again with the *ha-ha-ha* exhalation. Repeat this sequence five to seven times.

To properly carry out combined breathing, it is important to get to know the other two types of breathing: chest breathing and upper or collarbone breathing.

◥ Chest Breathing

1. Lie down on your back. Place your hands flat against your lower ribs.
2. Use the *ha-ha-ha* exhalation and close your eyes.
3. Now begin to inhale slowly through your nose, directly into your ribcage. This leads to a gradual expansion of the ribcage. Try to inhale only into your chest, not your abdomen. Focus your entire concentration solely on the ribcage. At the same time, use your hands to feel the space between the ribs expand.
4. Exhale slowly through your nose. Your ribcage will fall again and you can feel the loss of volume. Repeat this sequence five to seven times.

◥ Upper Chest or Collarbone Breathing

Pelvic breathing focuses on the bottom part, and chest breathing on the middle part of the lungs. But the tips of the lungs reach all the way up to the shoulders, and it is this upper portion of the lungs that is targeted during the exercise.

1. Lie down on your back and relax, or stand up, leaning forward slightly. Place your hands on your chest and your thumbs on your shoulders,

with your index fingers on the collarbone (the slightly protruding bone that connects the shoulders with the breastbone).

2. Close your eyes and begin the *ha-ha-ha* exhalation.
3. Breathe in slowly through your nose. Focus your attention on the upper part of your ribcage. Using your thumb and index finger, feel how your shoulders and collarbone rise solely because of your inhalation, not from lifting your shoulders. Now try to inhale into the very top of your lungs, and keep your attention focused on the upper part of your ribcage. This will oxygenate only the top part of your lungs. Relax while doing this.
4. Slowly exhale through your nose, feeling your collarbone and shoulders gently sinking. Repeat this sequence five to seven times.

❧ Combined Breathing

Once you have reached a level of comfort in carrying out pelvic, chest, and collarbone breathing and feel comfortable and confident in the exercises, you can begin with combined breathing.

1. Lie down on your back and relax. Place your hands next to your hips. Begin by moving your head, feet, and hands slightly back and forth, and then lie as still as possible.
2. Begin with the *ha-ha-ha* exhalation, causing your abdomen to fall, then breathe slowly and steadily through your nose. Consciously direct your breathing to your pelvis. Try to feel your pelvis down to the perineum and feel your abdomen rising. Count inside your head: one, two.
3. Continue breathing, now directing your breath into your ribcage; feel your chest expanding. Continue counting: three, four.
4. Continue breathing and focus your attention on the top part of your ribcage. Feel your collarbone and shoulders rise slowly. Count: five, six.
5. Exhale slowly and steadily through your nose. Repeat this sequence five to seven times.

❧ Alternate-Nostril Breathing

Inhaling through the right nostril connects us to our active, rational side, while inhaling through the left nostril connects us to our passive, emotional side. By inhaling through alternating nostrils, we can harmonize these contrasts within ourselves. This cleanses the main nadis, Ida and Pingala (see page 71), which allows for a better flow of life energy between the coccyx and brain.

1. Sit comfortably on a meditation cushion or a chair, holding your head upright and keeping your spine straight. Use the ring finger of your right hand to close your left nostril. Inhale and exhale a few times through your right nostril.
2. Now close your right nostril using the thumb of your right hand, and at the same time, remove your ring finger. Inhale and exhale through your left nostril for a few cycles.
3. Now begin with alternate breathing: inhale through the right nostril and exhale through the left nostril, opening and closing the nostrils as described above. You can relax your middle finger against your third eye (on the forehead between the eyebrows).
4. When you have exhaled through the left nostril, inhale through the left nostril, then close the left nostril with the ring finger, remove the thumb from the right nostril, and exhale through the right nostril.
5. That was one round. At the beginning, exercise for about five rounds, and then gradually increase the exercise to ten rounds.

⚘ The Tantric Breath of Fire

The Breath of Fire is a very powerful breathing exercise that stimulates life-force energy and concentrates it in our navel area at the third chakra. With this breathing technique, you can initiate a deep cleansing process that will pull toxins from the lungs and cells and deposit them into the bloodstream and lymph system, where they can be eliminated.

In addition to its strong effects on the lower body, the Breath of Fire also helps to:

- Cleanse the blood
- Remove toxins
- Improve circulation

Because of its strong cleansing effects, this exercise can sometimes cause nausea or dizziness. If these occur, it is important to rest, so that released toxins can be excreted. Drinking plenty of water supports the cleansing process. Women who have an IUD should not do this exercise, as it might cause the device to become dislodged. In the case of certain medical conditions, including circulation problems, bronchial problems, and heart arrhythmias, fire breathing should be done only after consultation with a doctor.

The Breath of Fire is fast and powerful, with the pause between inhalation and exhalation falling away. This should not be mistaken for panting, however, which would fill only the upper parts of the lungs. During this exercise, inhalation and exhalation occur through the nose; the shoulders remain relaxed and uninvolved. Practice this exercise with the window open to ensure that the room is filled with fresh air.

1. Sit down comfortably on a meditation cushion or a chair, keeping your head upright and your spine straight. Place one hand on your belly, and the other in the middle of your chest.
2. Prepare for this exercise by breathing quietly for two minutes and relaxing.
3. Take a deep breath, exhale two-thirds of the air slowly through your nose, then expel the rest with an active, forceful exhalation through your nose. While completing this exhalation, pull your belly quickly and sharply in toward your spine. The strength of the movement rapidly presses the diaphragm upward, pressing all of the air out of the lungs. Your mouth should be closed during exhalation, and the ribcage remains completely relaxed.
4. The inhalation that follows is purely passive; as you relax your abdominal muscles, the diaphragm that was pushed upward relaxes and lowers. Breath flows in completely quietly and without effort.

When done correctly, the Breath of Fire creates a rapid pumping movement of the diaphragm. In the beginning practice this exercise slowly, devoting one full second to each exhalation and one second to each inhalation. Then increase your pace so that you spend one second on the entire cycle (exhalation plus inhalation). Repeat ten to twenty times.

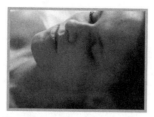

BREATHING DURING
YONI MASSAGE

Different cultures have different names and interpretations for life energy. In India it is called *prana,* in China *chi,* and in Japan *ki. Prana* and *chi* both mean "energy" as well as "breath," since traditional Indian and Chinese cultures both hold that life energy is inexorably linked to breathing and can be increased through certain breathing exercises.

Everything that we are able to do as human beings we owe to energy. The more energy we have, the more creative, mentally alert, and active we will be. The whole world, everything that exists, is wedded to this energy in the web of life. The energy flows in every cell of our body and streams through our meridians, which connect all parts of the body with one another. To distribute life energy, we can use the main energy cycle in our bodies—the Microcosmic Orbit discussed on page 66. It consists of the back channel (Governor Vessel) and the frontal channel (Conception Vessel). During yoni massage, sexual energy can be transmitted along the Microcosmic Orbit. From there, it flows into all meridians and supplies our entire being with energy.

A lot of sexual energy accumulates during yoni massage, which can be consciously used for transformation; we can channel this energy toward the expansion of consciousness, the revitalization of body and soul, and the achievement of greater flexibility and creativity. Using the breath and the powers of our imagination, we can circulate this new sexual energy throughout our bodies. The energy will follow our attention, which means that wherever we direct our mind, we will collect energy and increase the activity of nerves and muscles. The greater our concentration, the more energy is moved. The more we activate our breathing, the higher the degree of our sexual feeling and enjoyment.

ஃ Breathing in the Microcosmic Orbit

1. When sexual energy begins to flow during the course of the yoni massage, use your thoughts to send it upward along the spine/Governor Vessel as you inhale, and down the front/Conception Vessel as you exhale.

2. You can also use your PC muscle to support this exercise. Contract the muscle as you inhale, and use its contraction to send energy upward along the spine. Relax the muscle as you exhale, allowing energy to flow downward along the front of the body.

Along this channel (called Sushumna in India) lie our chakras, which become more relaxed and balanced with every breath. The flow of energy will have a different effect on each of the chakras, such that our emotions, thoughts, and feelings will change as the energy moves from chakra to chakra.

Breathing Phases during Yoni Massage

Just as the yoni massage progresses through several stages (see chapter 3), the intensity of our breathing also progresses through different phases during the course of the massage. There are four main breathing stages that can be practiced during a massage:

1. The first phase begins with deep pelvic breathing, which we use actively in the beginning, and to which we can revert throughout the yoni massage. This breathing forms the base from which all other breathing phases originate. It is often too overwhelming for women to use different breathing techniques during a massage. If that is the case, have the receiving woman focus simply on the deep pelvic breathing, and she can experience the sensations of the body through it.

2. In the second phase, we follow what author K. Ruby calls "filling breathing," which simply refers to a quicker and deeper pelvic breathing. This helps us to take in energy and activate it. This type of breathing often begins when the yoni flower begins to expand, which generates erotic sensations and indicates the beginning of sexual arousal. Inhalation and exhalation occur with the mouth

wide open but relaxed. Picture it as widening the body like a balloon and filling it with air, except that this time the breathing is quicker and more intense. This stimulates and charges every cell in the body, allowing us to reach a different level of consciousness and to enter into contact with the deepest core of our being. We become receptive and are able to accept touch in all its depth—not just the touch of massage, but touch overall, including the touch of subtle energies and the entire universe.

3. The third phase focuses on channeling the increasing sexual energy to make use of it physically and mentally. In this, we use our imagination to circulate the energy along the Microcosmic Orbit, allowing it to move throughout the body. This third phase of breathing can begin as soon as sexual energy is noticeably present. In some women this happens during stimulation of the pearl, while in others it happens only at the Goddess spot. It can also happen that a woman is not focused on her sexual energy and thus skips this phase.

4. The fourth phase is what Joseph Kramer has called the "Big Draw." This intense and effective breathing technique immediately follows the massage and often creates a trancelike conclusion. Through contractions of all body muscles, energy is bundled and then released to flow throughout the entire body.

The Big Draw

The Big Draw is used to distribute built-up energy throughout the body, so it doesn't remain confined to the genital area, where it may cause feelings to stagnate. This exercise is especially useful when a woman did not achieve orgasm but nonetheless reached a very high level of energy.

What happens in the Big Draw is physically and energetically very similar to orgasm. Because these two physical experiences are practically the same, the technique provides a way to climax without the commonly known orgasm. I initiate a Big Draw after orgasm only if the woman specifically requests it, which is rare.

In the Big Draw, the woman first exhales completely, then inhales fully and deeply. Then she tenses up her entire body: feet, legs, arms, stomach, shoulders, and face. She keeps this tension for as long as possible while also holding her breath, before exhaling and relaxing. Tensing the muscles this way elevates the arousal to a higher level. Then, when the muscles relax, the arousal of the nervous system falls quickly, much like a waterfall that cascades from a great height with enormous strength and then falls into a very deep and calm lake.

The most important point, however, occurs after the Big Draw, when the change in the nervous system causes energy to stream into the entire body, resulting in a calm akin to that reached in deep meditation. This is the moment when a woman can experience incredible peace and happiness. Between the Big Draw and this deep calm is a time of freedom, in which changes can manifest themselves.[4]

Usually people are very active during sexual interactions. But because the yoni massage involves only receiving, it invites us to enter a happy, peaceful, and calm space. After the Big Draw there frequently follow mystical experiences and visions. These experiences, which sometimes also occur during the yoni massage itself, are one of the reasons why this massage is so important. It offers us an opportunity to open our hearts and have a deep encounter with our entire being.

ℬ Experiencing the Big Draw

You are on your back. If you are highly aroused, then complete the following steps:

1. Exhale slowly and deeply, making sure to push all the air out of your body. This is best done by saying "fff" as you exhale. (If you have exhaled completely, you will experience a "hunger" for air, which will automatically cause you to inhale properly into your abdominal area.)
2. Take a deep breath.
3. Close your anus (as if you wanted to keep from defecating) and your throat, and hold your breath for at least one minute.
4. Then ball your hands into fists and tense all muscles as much as possible. If you would like, you can also pull your knees upward as you do this.
5. Hold, hold, hold . . .
6. And then let go. Relax completely and feel what is happening now inside your body.
7. If you wish, you can now mentally send this energy from your genital area to your heart.

If a woman's face becomes beet-red during the Big Draw, interrupt the exercise immediately! Otherwise, blood vessels in and around the head may burst, which could be dangerous. The next time she needs to place less tension in her head and neck and more in her anus, legs, and lower body.

The following is what women who practiced the Big Draw had to say:

- "It is a pleasant body exercise that generates heat and relaxes me."
- "Because I have breathing problems or sometimes forget to breathe, it felt good to have this experience. My whole body was flooded with energy."
- "I didn't have an orgasm during the yoni massage but was filled with sexual energy. Without the Big Draw, something would have been missing, and I would have felt unsatisfied. But the Big Draw helped me balance my energy. Afterward I no longer had the feeling that I desperately wanted to have an orgasm but felt filled with energy and eagerness to be active."
- "The energy is distributed in the whole body, the whole body is vibrating, and the light energy in the body is raised. I see a lot of light in the third eye and crown chakra. A flow or stream that engulfs the whole body."
- "The spirit is free and begins to flow—far beyond the body or deep within it, often connected with a deeper recognition of my own internal truths. Sometimes images appear from a previous life. Sometimes accompanied by feelings. Painful things from a previous life, but I experience healing, ending with a feeling: I can have joy again, be sexual, without being judged or shamed."
- "A pulsing in the whole body."
- "I practiced the Big Draw independent from massage, and it helped me be able to better use breathing to channel my sexual energy along the Microcosmic Orbit."
- "After the Big Draw I was able to flow in whichever direction I wanted to. It was a state that I don't even want to try to describe. It is the most complete state of happiness that I have ever experienced."

Erotic Trance

One of the most common feelings we have when energy begins to flow in our bodies is a strong pulsating or needling sensation. In some women this pulsating can build up slowly, while others experience it suddenly like a flood. Often, this energy also causes a slight twitching, warmth, or tickling. The sex researcher, theologian, and Taoist Dr. Joseph Kramer described this feeling as "erotic trance." He suggested that when a person enters into this erotic trance via breathing or erotic touch, he or she can reach a level of experience that is no longer connected to fantasies or behavior patterns. Rather, erotic trance connects us with the vibrations of the universe.

According to Kramer, people in an erotic trance enter a space of freedom and liberation. Their bodies know intuitively how to vibrate on this level to deepen the trance. These people reach a place where they are freed of limitations of any kind. They pass through a gate to places of healing, to other levels of consciousness, and to ecstasy.

For many women and for many reasons, sexuality is linked with fear. When they learn to breathe properly and thus reach a trance level during yoni massage, they may be able to let go of their fears and to integrate negative experiences such as sexual abuse.[5] The sex researcher, coach, and sex educator K. Ruby described the influence of breathing as follows:

> Breathing makes visible whatever is hiding below the surface. As long as we breathe automatically, we don't know what that is. Sometimes something comes up that was completely unexpected, and it may be so fundamental, important, and significant that one has to stay there. That is the moment that adds magic to massage. It is simply magical to be authentic with a woman, to be there for her, and to say, "Okay, we meant to go into your erotic experience, but here is something that's in the way, and we decide together to go just there." This process, to simply change direction when something else at that moment appears more important, is a very female energy. Whatever is visible, whatever happens—when we breathe, we emerge on the other side. With breathing we cannot stay still, it always carries on. Very often, on the other side we find ecstasy, joy, consciousness, or simply an "a-ha" moment. Sometimes on the other side we simply have appreciation of the blockade or pattern, but that too is an important step. Oftentimes

through touch and breathing we see blockades and patterns from a different perspective. This can help us to cross through them the next time, to be ready to transform that energy.[6]

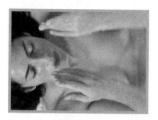

A BRIEF INTRODUCTION TO THE WORLD OF TANTRA

The yoni massage as we practice it at AnandaWave derives from a spiritual worldview based on tantric philosophy and Taoist techniques. Indian yoga culture, Native American shamanism, and Celtic knowledge also contribute essential elements to our practice.

Tantrism is a philosophical movement that accords central importance to human sexuality. With that belief, tantra developed a range of meditation techniques designed to enable people to use their sexual power for an internal transformation process. Tantrism is not a religion with dogmatic ideas, but rather an applied philosophy that embraces all aspects of life. It dispenses with confining societal structures in order to bring people into harmony with the bigger whole, to enable each person to experience the love and strength of the cosmos—the universal unity—within him- or herself.

The word *tantra* comes from the Sanskrit. Its root *tan* means "expanding," "thread," or "tissue." This refers to a large cosmic web in which we are all connected. Tantra unites opposites. Everything has two sides, and only when we recognize both of them without prejudices can we begin to understand the truth that lies behind them. In this way, we are confronted with situations and feelings in life that may appear pleasant or unpleasant, but every aspect of our experience wants to be felt and completely accepted, then transformed so as to allow its essence to appear.

In the tantric story of creation, the duality expressed by the male godly principle, Shiva, and the female godly principle, Shakti, plays a central role. While Shakti represents love and infinite empathy, Shiva represents Eros and mind. In this, Shiva and Shakti are seen not as fairy-tale characters, but as metaphors for the polarities of life. Together they represent a relationship of opposites in the cosmic web of creation.

Before the act of creation there was nothing other than the pure, shapeless being: Shiva and Shakti were one unit.[7] This pure, shapeless being was composed of a high-frequency, godly energy, pure consciousness, love, and light. In tantric philosophy, the great fulfillment is to experience this love and light; knowledge alone does not give us fulfillment. To experience love and unity, it is necessary for Shiva and Shakti to be able to recognize themselves as both linked and independent, solitary yet remaining unchanged as pure transcendent consciousness.[8]

In Western evolutionary history, this moment is called the big bang. From here, high-frequency energy flows into steadily changing material shapes and begins a never-ending process of evolution. In the tantric view, this process of energetic condensation—of manifestation—occurs in several steps. In our bodies, the shakti strength is manifested from top to bottom: first in the most subtle levels (seventh and sixth chakras), then in the different elements—ether (fifth chakra), air (fourth chakra), fire (third chakra), water (second chakra), and finally earth (first chakra).

Once embodied in the element of earth, the Shakti strength develops no further, and the creation process is complete. There, at the bottom of the spine, the Shakti power rests as latent energetic potential within us. This potential is called kundalini, and it is often depicted as a rolled-up snake. A central aim of tantric practitioners is to awaken the kundalini through a range of different techniques, and to have it rise through the chakras along the spine up to the seat of Shiva. According to tantric philosophy the kundalini carries the memory of unity with Shiva. This memory of pure consciousness, enriched and differentiated through the experience of duality, seeks a melting together and union. This desire is reflected in our search for spirituality, in our longing to be happy and whole.[9]

When the kundalini is awakened, whether through sexuality, a yoni massage, and/or different tantric techniques, it rises along the chakras through the channels (nadis) to Shiva, creating a different state of consciousness within us. This conciousness leads us back into the highest unity, the being beyond all polarities known as *samadhi*. In this state the never-ending dance continues between male and female, between Shiva and Shakti. It is a union of spirit with the manifestation of its godly form. In tantra, this

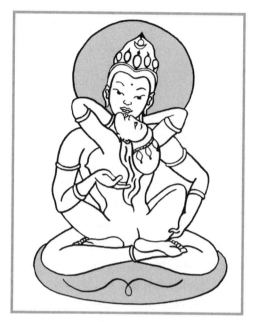

Fig. 2.9. The yab-yum position

union is depicted as Shiva and Shakti in an image of sexual union called the *yab-yum* position (see figure 2.9).

We all originate from a godly union and are connected to everything else. Earth, rocks, plants, and humans make up a living organism in the interplay of atoms, molecules, and cells. Everything is related, nothing exists separately or in isolation, everything is caught up in a highly developed web of life and consciousness. Like a big family, we are all connected to our surroundings by invisible ties; everything has its special place and its job to do. All our doing and thinking cause a reaction and an echo in the entire organism of life. That is what touches me so deeply in giving and receiving yoni massages, and what allows me to enter new and often unknown spaces with confidence and trust. I know that I am part of a larger whole.

Tantra invites us to recognize ourselves as Shiva and Shakti, as expressions of godly beauty and love. There is nothing in us that is not a part of this godly power. From this perspective, we can look at our "ugly" or "dark" sides anew, since in reality there is no darkness. Darkness is not a condition but, in the tantric sense, an absence of light. When we bring light to darkness, then hate turns into love, greed into generosity, ignorance into humility, and ugliness into beauty. The way of tantra is the way of love and the way of light. For that reason, I see this philosophy as the ideal spiritual frame for a yoni massage.

Tantric Massages

Tantra encompasses a wide variety of methods, techniques, meditations, and teachings whose essence is continually being reinvented. In this way, neo-tantrism has evolved into a tantra for people of our time and our culture. The form has adapted to our Western world, but the flower and scent of the original thought remain intact. The same can be said for well-founded tantric massages, which represent an important aspect of neo-tantrism.*

Truth cannot be found in the outside world. It is hidden in the body, which houses our deepest, innermost knowledge about the largest whole. The body is the temple of the soul, and it is for this reason that tantric practitioners approach the body with empathy, respect, and attention. Our massage work rests on the understanding that body, feelings, mind, and soul together form a whole. The goal of our work is to create a connection between spirituality, sensuality, and sexuality. For tantric practitioners, sexuality and spirituality belong together, as two sides of the same coin.

What is special about tantric massage and what differentiates it from other "alternative" types of massage is the conscious and concrete inclusion of the genital area, the yoni in the case of women and the lingam in the case of men. This allows a person to be accepted in his or her entirety, making sexual healing on a physical level possible. During tantric massage, people can find an oasis of calm, of relaxation, and of sensual ease. We work with the sexual chakra, the energy of which leads to the heart chakra, where it is transformed into love. Among some, an intuitive internal recognition of the godly power of unity appears. If that happens, nothing is ever the same again.

For those of us who give this massage, the meaning lies not only in what we do, but especially in how we do it. To massage an ordinary man, an ordinary woman, in the ancient spirit means to massage the god or goddess in a person. In this we see our tantric message.

---

*So-called tantric massages have become something of a fad, and there are many providers who use the term to mean prostitution. While we have no problem with prostitution, we consider true tantric massages to be only those that are carried out with tantric knowledge and in the tantric spirit.

3

The Yoni Massage

Parting

Gliding down into the depth
Between my legs
I rest
In the cave of the earth

Home
Of sadness

Home
Of desire

Calm
Pole of heat

My home
Is

The expansiveness in this place
Into which I stream
Conveying myself
Expansively
Into the depths
Between
All
Women's legs
Of this world.

—ANTONIA ALARIS

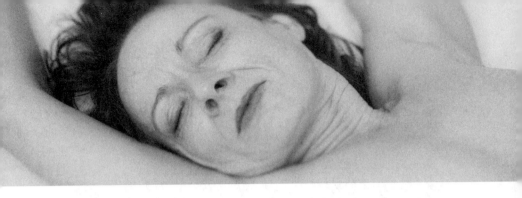

In the year 1995, I received my first yoni massage as part of a festive tantric ritual, which in turn was part of my tantric yoga training. Together with another twenty-two participants, I experienced this time of intense feelings in the impressive landscape of Tuscany.

I had some conflicting feelings during this time. On the one hand, I enjoyed the sun, the intensity, and the freedom to live to my fullest possible extent, but at the same time I felt clear reluctance and a great fear of my own sexual power. When I was supposed to receive my first yoni massage, I felt great curiosity and joy, but also a sense of inadequacy and great performance anxiety. Added to this were feelings of panic—I was afraid of feeling nothing at all, of being disappointed, and of disappointing my partner.

The choice of partner was very difficult for me. There was only one man with whom I could at that time consider carrying out this ritual. Although I knew that Silvio would be happy to do this kind of massage with me, I suddenly worried that he might choose somebody else. An otherwise rather hidden part of my personality emerged in the face of yoni massage and I suddenly felt very small, needy, and shy.

This experience made it very clear to me how important trust and security are; women need to be able to trust their partners before they can experience deep sexuality and the many releases associated with it.

While I did, finally, receive the yoni massage from Silvio, I was so exhausted by that point from various forms of tension that the first overwhelming feeling I had was simply one of letting go. This feeling was followed by a trust that I had never experienced before, along with an associated deep feeling of unconditional love.

What touched me at that moment was not that Silvio was using an effective technique, or that he was indeed a skilled masseur, but the fact that he gave me and my yoni his full presence in a ritualized way. It touched me deeply that he spent a full two hours with me, during which he was there only for me and my most intimate needs. In that moment, he gave me the best that he had to offer: his love and attention. His generosity gave rise to a deep peace and healing inside me, allowing the very effective techniques to work more deeply.

I immediately realized that the sexual injuries I had experienced on a physical level could be healed only on a physical level, and that I needed a loving and carefully protected space for this to happen. I experienced the complete yoni massage fully conscious and yet felt as if I were in a dream. I did not have an orgasm and instead carried out the Big Draw (see page 85). The resulting feeling is hard to describe: It was a kind of vibrating outside of myself, a feeling of being disconnected from all physical being, yet experiencing a strong physical presence. It was an intense dream state, combined with a clear and sharp perception of the here and now—a state of strong visionary strength and deep spirituality; a feeling of warmth, safety, and freedom.

I immediately knew that I wanted to give this special gift to as many people as possible, as a way of contributing a piece of healing to the world. At that time, the massage was the strongest experience of my life, and it had lasting effects on my sexuality. Since that time I cannot imagine my life or my relationships without yoni massage.

In 1998, I founded the women's research group Hysteria, with ten other women. (The group later changed its name to Dragon Trail.) We met four times a year for two or three intense days to explore and develop the significance of yoni massage on female sexuality. In this we used Native American and Celtic teachings, as well as tantric traditions.

In our attempts to understand the mysteries of femininity, we dealt very intensely with topics such as our bodies and our sexuality, menstruation and blood, hormonal cycles and the uterus, abuse and subtle energies, as well as initiation, masturbation, and sensual rituals. We embedded these topics into the experience of yoni massage. In exploring particular topics, experiencing a yoni massage helped us process many of our thoughts.

In all that we learned over the years, we learned especially that our internal readiness to fully immerse ourselves in the massage was a key point in its success. Whenever time pressures prompted us to try to quickly insert a yoni massage into the day, the attempt failed for one reason or another: one woman had a headache, another was too tired, the third needed fresh air, and so on. Good yoni massages occurred only when we had enough time to prepare, and enough time afterward to feel the effects of the massage.

We also found that all of us had difficulties expressing our intimate needs. Even though we were all dealing intensively with sexuality, almost all of us had great difficulties in clearly articulating what we needed in the realm of sexuality. We are formed by a social atmosphere that rejects women who openly discuss their sexual needs. We had to learn step by step to simply express our sexual desires and preferences. In this effort the yoni massages were and are a wonderful support.

I like to call yoni massages the "heart" of massages, since they offer access to a woman's most intimate area. In no other massage does a woman show as much of her personal and vulnerable side. With each yoni massage that I give, I develop deeper insight into the sensuality, tenderness, and significance of the female center.

The yoni has a receptive nature that corresponds to the female principle. For example, it receives the semen and all energies that are linked to it. Every sexual act and action for women means a complete opening of themselves, a reception of everything that happens in that moment. The woman receives and stores information in her yoni—information from personal experiences and from stories that have shaped entire generations of women. The yoni, the magical heart place, is thus home to many secrets, a place that recounts the smallest injuries and the greatest moments, as long as we can open its doors.

A person's different physical and emotional expressions reflect his or her relationship to the world. According to Wilhelm Reich, our muscle tensions are the reflection of our unprocessed experiences.[1] These blockages or physical tensions reduce our physical flexibility, our breathing, and the emotional intensity of our experiences. The intention of yoni massage is to resolve this information—these injuries, blockages, and memories—through targeted massage. In this, breathing has a central supporting role. The degree to which people are able to let go of their physical tensions increases with their ability to breathe freely, to give themselves over to spontaneous and unconscious movement impulses, and to experience their feelings in a more intense way. This can re-create space for joy, desire, and ecstasy.

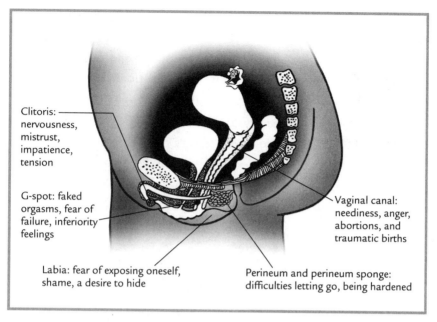

Clitoris:
nervousness,
mistrust,
impatience,
tension

G-spot: faked
orgasms, fear of
failure, inferiority
feelings

Vaginal canal:
neediness, anger,
abortions, and
traumatic births

Labia: fear of exposing oneself,
shame, a desire to hide

Perineum and perineum sponge:
difficulties letting go, being hardened

Fig. 3.1. Blockages in the yoni area

I see yoni massage as pioneering work that is helping to create a healthier society, one with friendlier attitudes toward sexuality, and one that does not deny our desire but celebrates it as the healthiest, most creative source of power that we have. Nothing, absolutely nothing, can open our hearts like and Eros and desire.

Even if the beginning of a yoni massage leads a woman through sadness and fear, the end always brings desire, joy, and happiness, as well as the orgasmic potential that makes intimacy possible. The word *intimacy* comes from the Latin and describes a state free of fear; in this sense, it is a state that can be reached only if we have the courage to encounter our fears.

The journey that yoni massage leads us through can cross many different terrains—deep canyons, but also the beauty of the world, the most tender love, waves of ecstatic arousal, and, finally, home into our own centers, into the cores of our being. In this way, the feelings that women have during a yoni massage can be very different, ranging from sadness, joy, anger, desire, and ecstasy to indifference, or a feeling that nothing is happening. Everything is allowed, and everything is correct. Every feeling tells its own story, which unfolds as it receives the necessary attention, which finally allows it to leave us forever.

The yoni massage offers the space to discover and explore our own sexuality without performance pressure or expectations. Attention focuses on recognizing what there is. Like a mother who simply observes her child at play, a woman during the yoni massage notes all feelings and emotions without judging or influencing them. This judgment-free space is what makes a rediscovery of our own femininity possible.

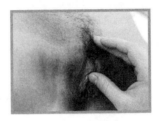

THE REFLEXOLOGY ZONES OF THE YONI

Just like our feet, hands, and ears, our yonis have reflexology zones that are linked to certain organs. This is why stimulation of the yoni creates such a pleasant feeling throughout the body. In men, the lingam has the same reflexology zones in exactly the reverse order (see figures 3.2 and 3.3). When the lingam penetrates deep into the yoni, these reflexology zones rest on top of one another, a contact through which they stimulate and harmonize each other. Nature could not have arranged things more perfectly. For me, this is once again proof that sexuality between a man and a woman not only serves reproductive purposes but is also a key to our health and vitality.

In yoni massage, these reflexology zones are treated extensively. The massage loosens the shield of the entire yoni, freeing the muscles of the pelvic floor, which then allows for more flexibility and pleasure in lovemaking. The energy centers of the body are harmonized and strengthened, allowing women to emerge from the massage relaxed and empowered.

During yoni massage, the raw sexual energy, termed *ching* in Chinese, is converted into fine energy, or *chi*. The *ching* is stored at the

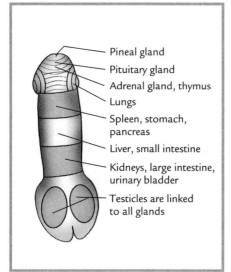

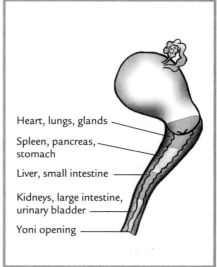

*Fig. 3.2. The reflexology zones
of the lingam*

*Fig. 3.3. The reflexology zones
of the yoni*

lower end of the spine. It is this energy that is stimulated and heated during yoni massage and that rises up along the spine by the end of the massage, to be distributed throughout the entire body. Focused breathing along the Microcosmic Orbit (see page 84) can support and intensify this process.

Before administering a massage, I often ask women what needs, expectations, and pictures they have of the upcoming treatment. In this way, I can sense what specific themes are currently at the forefront of their thoughts. Should it be a journey that focuses on loosening the pelvic floor and massaging the muscles around the yoni to stimulate circulation? Or should it be a gentle, calm yoni massage that leads to places of internal peace and invites a woman to let go? Or is there a way to strengthen the joyful and erotic tendency of yoni massage to express the orgasmic potential? Or, yet again, should the focus be on breathing, to increase the body's sexual sensitivity and reach an erotic trance?

Arousal during yoni massage usually follows a wavelike cycle, and its energetic results run through many phases. It may be useful to begin with an idea of an approximate goal that the massage is aiming toward.

But whatever the needs or wishes of the woman are, it is important to know that these can change at any moment. It may be that her body's signals will point in a different direction. For that reason, the person giving the massage needs to be fully present during each moment, to ensure that the signs and reactions of the woman's body are reflected in the massage.

Once I gave a yoni massage to a woman who felt sadness and pain from the outset. I was mainly attempting to hold the woman and carry out only slow and careful movements, feeling reasonably sure that this pain and sadness would be the only themes of this massage. But at one point those energies began to decrease, and when I was about to finish the massage a completely different energy unfolded from the yoni. I followed this energy; my movements quickened and became more intense, the woman's breathing quickened, and then her pelvis began to vibrate by itself. Finally, the massage ended in a very deep orgasm. We were both completely surprised. We had followed her body's energy and language, which at that moment had decided to transform the pain into joy.

I often also experience these energy changes in the reverse sequence. Very joyful moments can suddenly transform into sadness, anger, and despair, since these energies in some women stand in the way of desire and joy. Sexuality is a mirror of our emotions: it brings all themes of our personality into view.

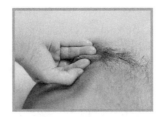

THE YONI MASSAGE—PHASE BY PHASE

Every yoni massage is unique and can be a new experience even for the same woman. In giving or receiving a yoni massage, we always enter a place of unknowing, which demands of us complete surrender to the here and now.

In the following section I describe the yoni massage in some detail.

The sequence of the individual steps, however, should be seen as a suggestion only. It would not be in the spirit of yoni massage to stick to this sequence too strictly. I view the phases that make up the arc of the journey of yoni massage as more important than the individual steps. It is the individual phases that appeal to the wholeness of a woman. For this reason, it makes more sense to concentrate on the individual phases than on a program that is locked in every detail. There is no right or wrong. The only things that count are the well-being and trust of your partner. She and the energy of her body determine the individual steps.

A clear and protected framework is a precondition for the journey of discovery that we undertake during a yoni massage. The room should be clean and well kept, since external order also creates internal order. Fresh flowers, pleasant scents, candlelight, lovely music, and nice fabrics quickly turn an ordinary room into a sensual oasis. The room must be pleasantly warm (at least 82 degrees F) and must be protected against sudden interruptions. This assurance of privacy allows the woman to concentrate completely on herself and thus opens the possibility for her to trust, give in, and let go. The massage should last for at least one and a half hours, and two hours if possible.

During the massage, the giving person and the receiving person do not enter into a sexual relationship. This is very important, since only in this way can the receiving woman take the space necessary for her journey. The otherwise common internal questions like "How is the other person feeling? Is he/she receiving enough? Am I too egotistical? Am I allowed to be pleasured for this long?" can be precluded through clearly defined roles, in this case establishing one person as the giver and the other as the receiver.

Each yoni massage should be preceded by a ritual honoring the woman in her entirety and by a full-body massage. The honoring of femininity (Shakti) and the honoring of masculinity (Shiva) are of great importance in tantra, since they express a respect for all living things. This honoring creates trust in the receiving person. At the same time, the full-body massage ensures that the person is fully comfortable in her body.

I will not go into extensive tantric full-body massage techniques, since that would go beyond the scope of this book. Instead, I will discuss a few simple, easily applicable ideas that can be implemented with joy and ease. They are ideas and suggestions—they do not aim to set limits to the imagination, and nothing has to be done exactly as it is described here.

Erotic and empathetic touch are less matters of well-practiced technique than they are matters of love, presence, and devotion. Eroticism is always a game of contrasts, a balance of different strengths: tension and relaxation, tender and strong touch, the alternation between the known and the new. Whatever joy, lightness, relaxation, and depth we are able to summon when giving the massage is what we will pass on to the person receiving it.

Before the Massage

We are all full of images and ideas about sexuality. We are used to slipping into sexual roles and experiencing our desire in a very specific framework. We are used to thinking of ourselves as a girlfriend or a wife, a mistress or a whore, passive or active, in love or simply after sex. Every woman develops certain sexual behavior patterns, even during masturbation.

It is important to let go of these ideas and images. Only then do we truly create a space that allows us to experience new aspects of our sexuality and expand our notions of what sexuality can be. For many women this is an immense challenge, and the yoni massage can be a great help in achieving this openness. It invites women to simply do nothing for a change, to inhale deeply, and to dive into new bodily sensations. The goal is not an orgasm, but an orgasmic mind. The orgasm is a welcome side effect, but the intent of the yoni massage is a simple recognition of what happens, without any expectations attached.

In the process of yoni massage, the giver lights a fire in the clitoris of the receiver, and this fire must be nourished throughout the massage— sometimes more and sometimes less. It is thus important to stimulate the clitoris once in a while and not lose sight of it completely during certain moves. At the same time, be careful to avoid overstimulation—your touch on the clitoris must not be too strong and must always be done with enough lubricant. It is also good to include breaks in the stimulation, for example when focusing on a different part.

This report from a woman whose clitoris was not touched at a certain point in her massage shows us the importance of this work. "That feels a bit like being abandoned," she said. "Perhaps that is because the energy created by the stimulation of the clitoris is more 'male.' It feels like guys that no longer look after me. Somehow it is important for me that the clitoris is incorporated, even if it is just a gentle stroking over it, that would be enough."

There are many different ways to massage a yoni, with no general statement that applies to all women in the same way. Every yoni massage is a great adventure and the path is always new; there is no set direction. Instead, the direction follows from the flow of the massage and the signals of the Shakti energy. However, because many women have forgotten how to give clear signals, this is sometimes not easy.

Do not be discouraged if at first things don't go the way you had hoped. There will always be several moments in a yoni massage that demand a certain clarity of direction. The possibilities, however, are many, and it is always an art to find the right moment and the right path. Do not expect to always do the right thing, because that expectation is sure to lead to disappointment. The yoni and female sexuality are both too complex for easy answers. Approach yoni massage with an open, curious, aware, and loving attitude, and see what you can learn from this woman. She will show you the way. When you reach a point on the path that is unclear, you can ask the Shakti for guidance. You will learn a lot that way.

As masseuse or masseur, you are there to serve and accompany. Your goal is to support and serve the wishes of the Shakti—it is her journey. Your own wishes, needs, and expectations need to be put aside for the duration of the massage. Especially once you have a lot of experience, you will quickly be able to intuit what the body of the Shakti needs. It is nonetheless a good idea to ask before suddenly changing direction, for instance by saying, "Can I touch you like this now?" or "I'm going to try something now, and if it doesn't work for you, please tell me." This gives the woman the assurance that you are not simply doing with her what you want, but that you continue to let her make the decisions.

To a woman who receives the yoni massage, I want to say this: Assume that the person giving you the massage is giving you the best he or she can. Accept this gift with love, and if something doesn't go as you want, have patience and show your partner the way. Nobody can guess your wishes; you have to learn to show them.

❧ *Phase 1: Honoring the Shakti*

The first phase creates an atmosphere that supports the letting go necessary for a successful yoni massage. It is dedicated to honoring the receiving woman, whom we also refer to as Shakti. Women can let go completely only when they feel well and safe; our sexuality is primarily a question of trust.

For that reason, the yoni massage begins with a welcoming and appreciative gesture from the giver. For this, a beautiful space is created that the giving and receiving persons now enter together. In a comfortable massage area, sit down across from one another, wearing a nice kimono, bathrobe, or sarong (body-length cloth). It is best if the giving person gives clear directions: "Please sit down" is always better than "Would you like to sit down?" since the latter automatically prompts consideration, thinking, and insecurity.

1. Make eye contact with the receiving woman, and take in her character. This is easier if you look into her left eye, since this mirrors her emotional side.
2. Give her your left hand with your palm facing upward and say, "Please give me your hand." The receiving woman then places her right hand into your left hand, with her palm facing down.

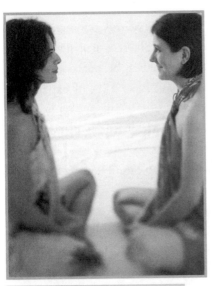 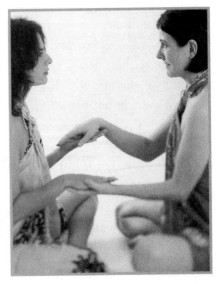

Phase 1: Honoring the Shakti

3. Now say, "Then I give you my hand," and offer your right hand with the palm facing down. The receiver offers her left hand beneath yours, with her palm facing up. You lower your right hand into hers. In this way, a cycle of giving and taking is created between the two of you.

4. With your hands touching, offer an invitation. For example: "I invite you to this sensual journey into the center of your femininity and will give you my best, so that you can fully trust and give yourself to the moment. For the duration of the massage, I will be there only for you, for everything that you need. When you are ready for the massage, please pull back your hands."

5. Now bring your hands into the motion of prayer and bow to each other.

6. Say, "Please stand in front of me." Then stand up and show your partner with a hand motion where you would like her to stand, and stand facing her at a comfortable distance. Now see her in her entirety and beauty.

7. Begin to spin a "tantric thread of luck" around her. Symbolically, you are using this to connect Heaven with Earth, which for Tibetans is a magical union of the spiritual with the earthly. Begin with the right shoulder and circle her body with your right palm, making a downward spiral until your hands reach her feet.

8. Place your hands on her feet, kneel down in front of her, and bow. This symbolizes the honoring of her temple, her godliness. In our Western world, such a position of humility is often mistaken for submission.

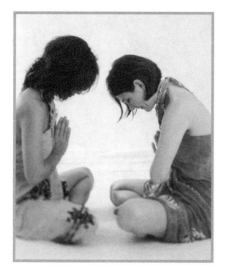 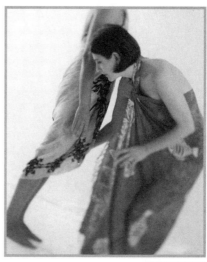

Phase 1

But only an emperor is able to bow with humility and recognition before his people, a gesture that demonstrates true strength, courage, and character. This is one of the most powerful and important gestures that one person can give to another. You can now also say an internal prayer, for example one from the Sanskrit: "*Om namah Shakti*—I honor everything godly in you."

9. Now is the time to disrobe your partner. In this, it is important to celebrate the disrobing with care and enjoyment, without hurry. Slowly undo the knot of the kimono or sarong, then slide your fingers under the fabric and push the kimono or sarong away from the shoulders. Stand behind your partner and slowly take off her kimono. Treasure each touch of the kimono to her naked skin, and play a little with this. Then neatly place her kimono to the side.

10. Stand behind your partner and use your touch to describe the energy cycle of her body. First gently stroke the spine/Governor Vessel upward. With your hands flat, stroke and touch her entire back from the top downward, along the outside of her legs down to her feet. Stroke along

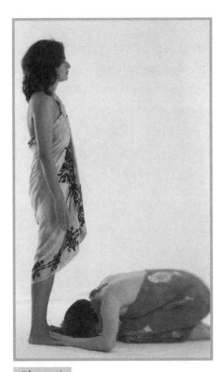
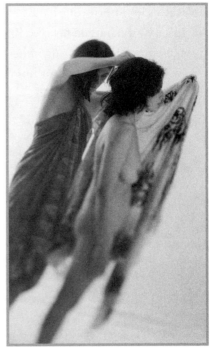

Phase 1

the feet, then run your hands along the inside of the feet and up along the inside of the legs, through the pelvis, and across the stomach to up between the breasts. Now continue up across the armpits and along the insides of the arms, along the palms, and on to the fingertips. Move your hands again and stroke from the outside across the fingers, along the back of the hands, along the outside of the arms, and up to the shoulders. Carefully glide up the throat and face. Then return downward via the entire back, until you are once again at the outside of the legs and down by the feet. Begin anew and repeat this about three times.

11. Now gently push up against your partner from behind and place your right hand on her lower abdomen and your left hand on her heart. Make sure you are standing firmly to allow the Shakti in front of you to be able to lean back against you without falling. From here, you can say after a while: "Please lie down on your stomach, with your arms next to your body." With this, you begin the massage on her back (yang side).

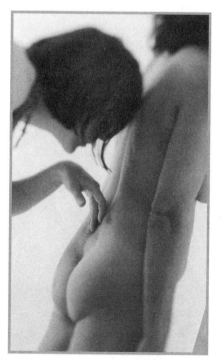
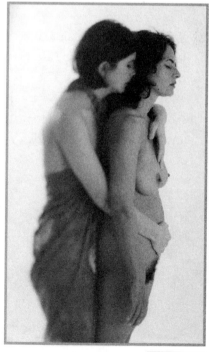

Phase 1

❀ *Phase 2: The Preparatory Full-Body Massage*

From the honoring and appreciating of the first phase, we continue with the second phase, a full-body massage to set the mood. In this phase, the most important thing is to observe and see this woman with love. By touching her entire body, you will give your partner a feeling of acceptance that will allow her to open herself to sexual and erotic energies. This creates the foundation that will carry the Shakti through the entire experience of her massage and will give her the most important feeling—that of being fully recognized.

The breathing in this phase is rather quiet and should go deep down to the pelvic floor.

❧ Massaging the Yang Side

Your partner is now lying on her stomach.

1. Sit behind her head and take off your clothes, as slowly and sensually as you previously removed hers. Take your sarong or another nice cloth, and gently place this on your partner's head. Now go down to her feet and from there pull the cloth across her whole back, making slight wave movements. Pull the cloth across her feet and steadily pull it from her body.

2. With a feather, touch and stroke the entire back of your partner in long, gentle strokes. Alternate between playful, quick strokes and slower, lingering ones. The most important thing in this is to touch the body evenly all over. To vary the feeling you can also turn the feather around and use the quill to make light touches, or use fur, your hair, or any kind of erotic accessories.

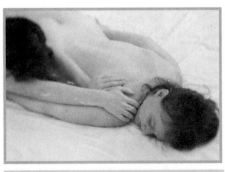

Phase 2: Massaging the Whole Body

3. Use your fingertips to touch her whole body. Here too you can alternate between a very slow touch and a somewhat faster one, thus creating an erotic and varied tension. What's important is that you are enjoying the touch, so that your joy will transfer to your Shakti.

4. Take a little oil and gently spread it in slow strokes across her entire body. A base oil is best for this—I recommend almond oil, sesame oil, or jojoba oil. Let your hands flow like waves, and have them slide over her body steadily. Make sure to keep your wrists loose, so that your touch is gentle and soft on the skin.

5. Sit at your partner's head and massage both halves of her back in circling movements, from the head down to the buttocks, beginning at the spine and moving outward. Continue along the sides of the body with wavelike movements back up. Include the shoulders and neck in this massage.

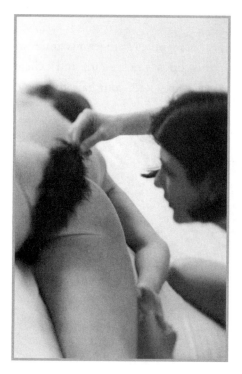
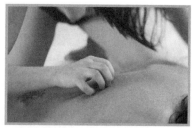
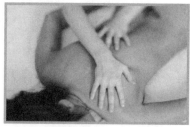
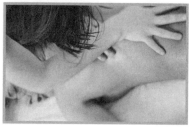

Phase 2

6. Sit down to the right of your partner. With flowing and kneading movements, massage her right arm from the shoulder down to the fingertips. Massage her hand, then each individual finger, beginning with the thumb and continuing on to the pinkie finger. Picture yourself pulling tension, bad thoughts, blockages, and so on from her fingers, then repeat the same on her other side.

7. Knead both of your partner's buttocks, from the inside upward and outward.

8. Now massage the entire right leg from the hip down to the feet with flowing movements. Repeat the same with the left leg.

9. Place your hands on the soles of her feet. Rest there for a while, then say to your partner, "Please turn over."

ᴄᴤ Massaging the Yin Side

Your partner is now lying on her back.

10. Touch and stroke the front of your partner's body with a feather, just as you did earlier with her back.

11. Caress her body with your hair and blow on the erogenous zones of her navel, nipples, and neck. For this, open your mouth and exhale with a long and deep "Haaa." Stroke her face with your hair and come to a rest behind her head.

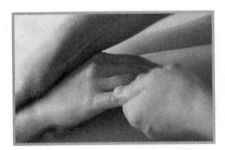

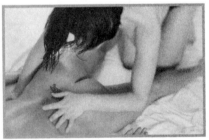

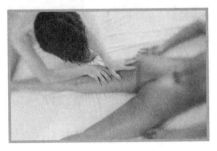

Phase 2

12. Now apply a scented oil to her erogenous zones, making circling movements at individual spots: the indentation of her neck, the beginning of the armpits, inside the elbows, and inside the wrists, then the palms, nipples, navel, pelvic region, backs of the knees, and inside the ankles. At each spot, place an impulse, as if you were throwing a stone into water and were taking the time to watch the resulting ripples until the surface of the water returns to rest. For the scented oil you can use a few drops of rose, jasmine, ambra, geranium, or ylang ylang (making sure they are accepted by your partner's skin), mixed into a base oil, for example almond or jojoba oil.

13. Now take a fan and fan the scent of the air toward her nose.

14. Carry out a massage using your fingertips on the front yin side, just as you did on the back yang side.

15. Sit down at your partner's head and take her hair and play with it—pull it gently, reach into it, then gently massage her scalp.

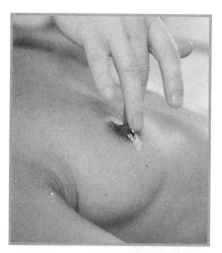
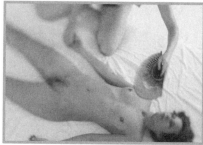
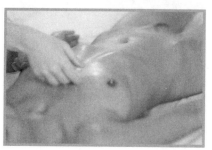
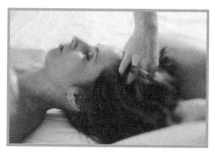

Phase 2

16. Pour some scented oil into your hand and gently spread it on her face, making sure that no oil runs into her eyes. With your slightly oily hands, stroke the face, beginning from the center and moving outward to the ears. Use the tips of your thumbs to massage her face, from the center outward and from the top down. Massage the temples, the nose, and the area around the mouth, letting each of your movements end at the ears.

17. Pour oil into your hand and spread it across her chest and stomach. Sit as close to her head as is comfortably possible for you.

18. Massage her front by stroking down the center of her body from the throat to the pubic bone, returning back up along the outside edge of her body and across the armpits, shoulders, neck, and head.

19. Sit on your partner's left side and massage or circle her breasts by making an upward/outward circle around them from the center of the body. From there, continue to circle over the shoulders and down the arms and massage them.

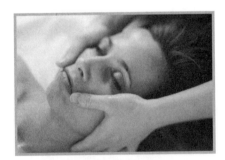

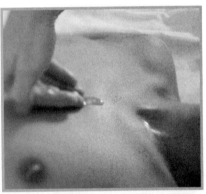

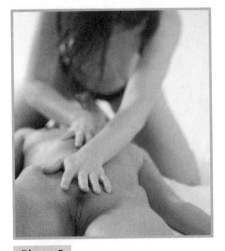

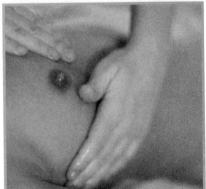

Phase 2

20. Very gently massage her stomach in clockwise motions (the natural cycle of the digestion).

21. Massage her left leg from the hip down to the feet. Repeat the same with her right leg.

22. Take both feet at the heels and pull her legs, then lightly move her feet back and forth to gently vibrate her whole body.

23. Now place the soles of her feet against your stomach. If her feet are very cold, you can heat your hands by rubbing them against each other. Breathe deeply to allow your partner to feel your breath on her feet.

24. Place your partner's legs far enough apart that you are later able to begin the yoni massage. Be very careful and aware, since by opening the legs you are also opening the innermost part of your partner. This opening must never cross her limits, making it important to take seriously even the smallest amount of resistance, which might indicate that your partner needs a little more time.

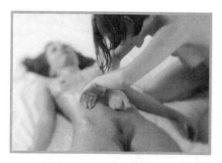
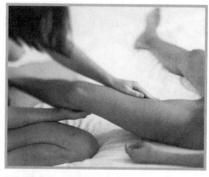
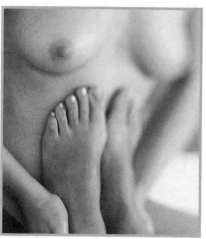
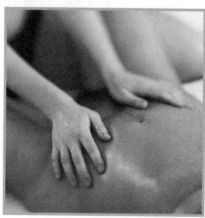

Phase 2

✿ *Phase 3: Awakening Desire*

The third phase is very significant for female sexuality. The giver includes particularly sensitive parts of the body in the massage while remaining in an accepting and loving state. The path of touch continues, making the connection from heart to yoni, energetically recharging the ovaries and uterus, and playfully tugging on the pubic hair, thus waking erotic feelings. Specifically, include the sensitive areas of the receiving woman, such as the neck, breasts, face, area between the legs (but not the yoni), fingers, and toes.

In this phase too the breathing is rather quiet but can quicken at times. It remains important that the breathing is deep, reaching down to the pelvic floor.

1. **Heart-genital touch:** Rub your hands against each other until they are hot, and then place your left hand on your partner's heart and your right hand on her yoni. Massage the canal in between. In this way, you create a connection between heart and sexuality. Charging the second and fourth chakras is the energetic focus of yoni massage.

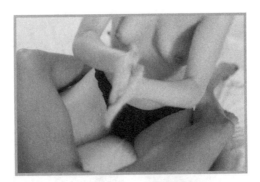

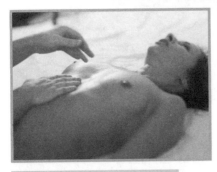
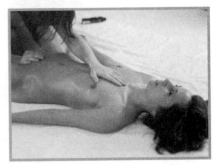

Phase 3: Awakening Desire

2. **Ovary warmer:** Rub your hands against one another until they are hot and charged, then place both your palms over your partner's ovaries. This wakens the sexual energy, which the Chinese call *ching chi.*
3. **Uterus warmer:** Place your two hot and charged hands over the uterus. This too wakens the *ching chi.* Playfully tug the pubic hair.

⚜ Phase 4: Opening the Yoni Flower

K. Ruby calls the fourth phase the "opening of the yoni flower." The purpose here is not a direct stimulation, but an observation and excitement of the entire yoni. It is touched and discovered from the outside, playfully circled, vibrated, and knocked on. The labia are massaged extensively. There is a lot that can happen in this phase—the goal is to awaken erotic feelings and to open the yoni. During this phase the body is very willing to send messages and express where the journey should lead. The breathing, which continues to go deep to the pelvic floor, may slowly intensify.

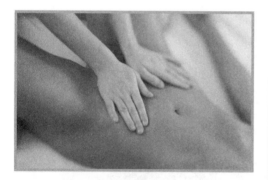
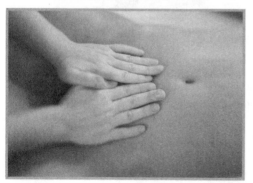
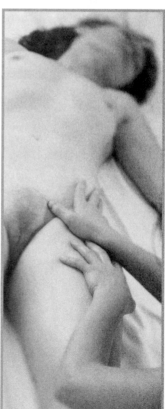

Phase 4: Opening the Yoni Flower

1. **Tapping:** With your hands and fingertips, gently tap on the genital region from the sacral bone (sliding your hands slightly under the buttocks) to the yoni hill. Include the inside of the thigh in this, and try to find a steady rhythm, as if playing a drum.

2. **Vibrating:** Cover the yoni with your right hand, so that the ball of your hand touches the clitoris. Let your hand vibrate a little, so that it lightly stimulate the clitoris. The other hand connects the different chakras by moving in a wavelike way from chakra to chakra. Only very few massage therapists are able to reach the head chakras from a seated position, but this touch can be intended. In this way, the channel from the earth chakra to the head chakra is stimulated. Energy can flow more easily, and the chakras are cleansed. This exercise is well liked, since it generates feelings of safety, warmth, energy, and protection. Press the outer labia together using both thumbs, pressing deep into the tissue. From the top move downward in intervals of one thumb width.

3. **Outer labia:** Apply plenty of nonscented lubricant to the entire yoni. Pull out one of the outer labia and massage it gently from the inside

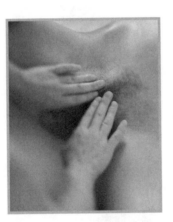
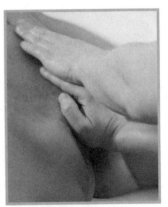
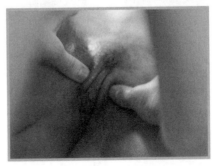

Phase 4

up and from the outside down, using your thumb and index finger. Then massage the other outer lip in the same way.

4. **Inner labia:** Gently pull out one of the inner labia and massage it—up the inside and down the outside, using your thumb and index finger. Then do the same with the other inner lip.

5. **Circling the Venus lips:** With your middle finger between the inner and outer labia, make circling movements from the perineum to above the clitoris and back down again.

6. **Lighting a fire:** Rub the inner labia with both index fingers, keeping your fingertips pointed downward. This motion will gently stimulate the clitoris. The clitoris will feel like a pea between your fingers; feel free to play with it.

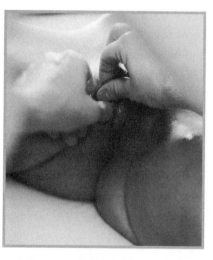
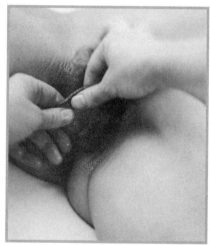
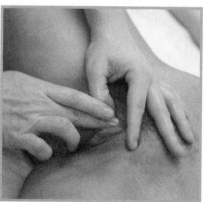
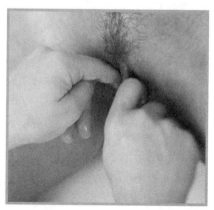

Phase 4

✖ *Phase 5: Stimulating the Pearl*

The fifth phase is what I call "stimulating the pearl." It begins with a very careful approach to the clitoris and ends with direct stimulation of it. This phase can be marked by a very strong flow of erotic energy, with some women already experiencing orgasm at this stage. However, I often try to avoid this, so that the woman can experience a more holistic feeling of arousal. The principle is not to break the wavelike building of sexual energy. On the other hand, for some women an orgasm in this early stage is exactly right.

In this as in the following phases, it is important to include the rest of the body every once in a while. During this phase, breathing may become deeper and quicker. You can encourage your partner to circulate her breath along the Microcosmic Orbit, as described on page 84.

1. Begin with a gentle touch and tickle of the clitoris.
2. With your index finger or thumb, draw small, gentle circles around the clitoris. This is a very well-liked form of clitoral stimulation.

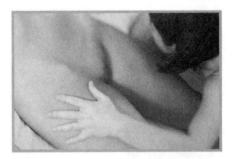

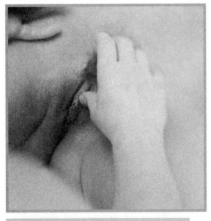 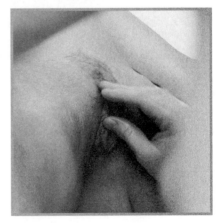

Phase 5: Stimulating the Pearl

3. Gently tug and pull the clitoris.
4. Using your thumb and index finger, pull the hood back and forth.
5. Massage the clitoris in whichever way your partner likes. Just ask her!

Every now and again, distribute the energy across the whole body. Massage the abdomen, breasts, arms, and legs. Touch the toes, fingers, and face. Gently rock the entire body by shaking it lightly.

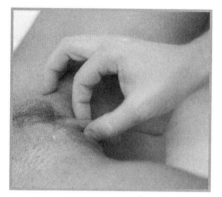
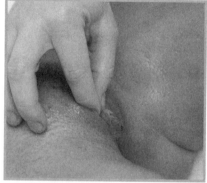

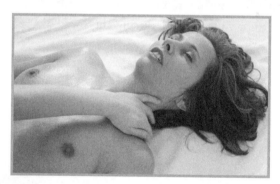

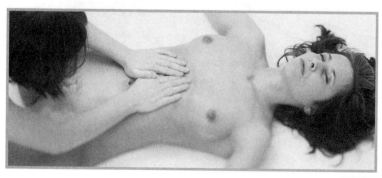

℘ Phase 6: Entering the Temple

The sixth phase is what I call "entering the temple." Here, inside the yoni, each woman has a very unique space. Are the mountains low or high? Are the valleys wide or narrow? How do the skin, the walls, the muscles, the skin flaps feel? What are the temperature and moisture levels?

This phase can be very emotional because a lot of information is stored inside the yoni. In this sense, the yoni is like a memory center that stores events that may have occurred years ago and may have been repressed inside us. Such memories can return to the surface when we "enter the temple."

Touching the yoni on the inside requires a high level of alertness from the giver, but also from the receiving woman. It is very important to focus on breathing, since this will prevent a "dreaming away" (getting lost in one's thoughts) and will instead continuously redirect the receiver's attention to the feelings in her body. Emotions, blockages, colors, and scents can be brought to consciousness more directly through mindful breathing. This particular phase of the yoni massage is usually quieter, as the energy deepens and spreads. Since the preceding phase of stimulating the pearl was intensely arousing, most women will still want their clitoris to be stimulated from time to time during the internal exploration of the yoni.

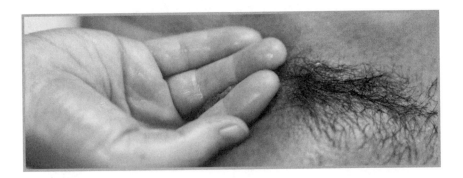

Phase 6: Entering the Temple

1. **Entering the temple:** Ask your partner for her permission to enter the inside of her yoni. In this, it is important to phrase the question in such a way that your partner only has to answer with yes or no. For example: "Is it alright if I now slide my finger into your yoni?" Use plenty of lubricant for this.

2. **Drawing in:** Place your finger on the yoni gate and wait for the yoni to open itself and let you inside. If she wishes, your partner can carry out the PC exercise at this point (see page 23) and actually draw your finger inside her.

3. **Four directions:** Massage the entire yoni from the inside with slightly circling movements. For this, picture the yoni as the face of a clock. Twelve o'clock points upward toward the clitoris and six o'clock downward toward the anus. Begin at twelve o'clock and use light circling

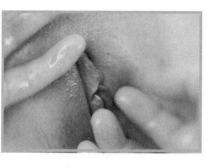
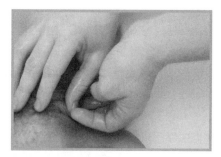
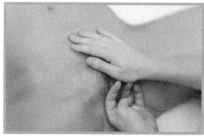
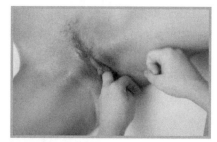
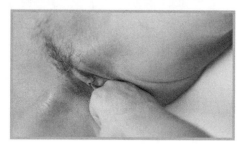

movements to move from back to front, then move around the clock in "five-minute" increments until you return to twelve o'clock. In this way, you will be sure to reach every part of the inside of the yoni.

This is the most emotional part of the yoni massage. It is important to give yourself plenty of time for this phase. Often there are small areas that suddenly become very hot, or areas in which small knots have formed. Oftentimes, negative information is stored in these areas. It is best to simply rest your finger on these spots and make only very small circling movements, if any at all. Sometimes the heat will fade away, and the knots may resolve themselves. Intense feelings, images, or scents may surface for the woman receiving the massage,

Phase 7: Stimulating the Goddess Spot

The seventh phase, which I call the "Goddess spot," also takes place inside the yoni, but it is more about stimulation than it is about the exploration that took place in the previous phase. In this phase the G-spot is discovered and stimulated. A touch that alternates between the clitoris and the G-spot makes this phase a holistic, arousing, and intense experience. This is the energetic high point, and the phase in which a woman is most likely to reach orgasm.

The powerful stimulation will lead to an intensification and quickening of the breath. Some women, however, will instinctively hold their breath at this point in reaction to the high level of tension. The giver can support the Shakti by recognizing the stop in breathing and gently accompanying her as a way of restarting her breathing. If the woman wants to, she can use her imagination to circulate this high energy once again in the Microcosmic Orbit, though for some women this is too much at this point in the massage.

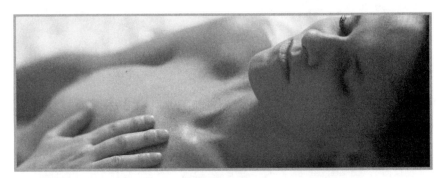

Phase 7: Stimulating the Goddess Spot

1. **Locating the G-spot:** In most women, this highly erogenous zone is located in an area about an inch inside the yoni, slightly to the left from the perspective of the giver, in the upper front part of the yoni canal. This Goddess spot rests in a small indentation that feels slightly ribbed, while the surrounding area is smooth.

2. Massage the entire G-spot area gently in circling movements, using one or two fingers and making sure to apply a steady amount of pressure.

3. Now "ring" the G-spot like a bell, by pressing and letting go, pressing and letting go, with varying amounts of pressure.

4. Stimulate the G-spot with zigzag movements and by gently sliding your fingers into and out of the yoni (the latter is usually preferred). At the same time, use your thumb or index finger to stimulate the clitoris.

5. Continue to alternate between G-spot simulation, clitoris stimulation, and a simultaneous stimulation of the two.

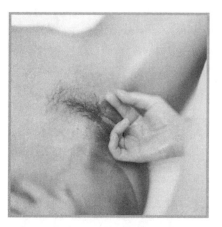
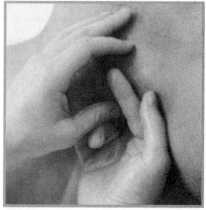
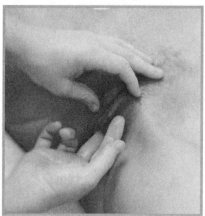
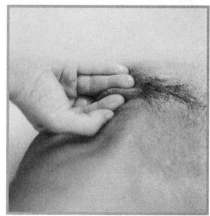

Phase 7

6 **Three-finger technique:** Use your middle finger to slide in and out of the yoni, while your index and ring fingers glide up and down the outer and inner labia, thus stimulating the clitoris resting between them.

7. **Three-finger combinations:** Let one hand carry out the three-finger technique, while the other hand massages the breasts, shoulders, neck, thigh, et cetera.

8. **Sprinkle/Kramer maneuver:** The thumb of your right hand glides into the yoni, while the fingers of your left hand stimulate the clitoris. Stimulate the G-spot and clitoris, sometimes alternating, sometimes simultaneously.

9. **PC exercise:** Guide the receiver to contract and relax her PC muscle, then to press the PC muscle outward, as if forcing something out of her yoni. During very high arousal these exercises can lead to a female ejaculation during this phase of the massage.

10. **The softener:** Use one, two, or three fingers to penetrate the yoni, while at the same time turning the hand and moving it in and out—very gently or strongly. You can use the fingers of the other hand to stimulate the clitoris at the same time.

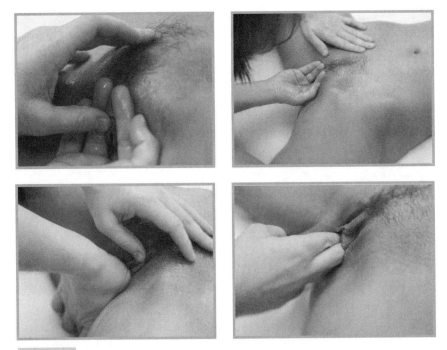

Phase 7

🎐 Phase 8: The Finale

The eighth phase is what Annie Sprinkle and Joseph Kramer call the "finale." The goal of this phase is to slowly calm the energy and to have the partner anchor herself again. The energy level in the receiver slowly ebbs, while energy is held, calmed, and distributed. The gates are lovingly closed. For women who did not experience an orgasm, this is the time to practice the Big Draw.

1. **The cervix:** With the pelvic floor relaxed, it is now possible to touch the cervix. Slide two fingers deep into the yoni and search for the cervix. The exact location will vary from woman to woman, and also depends on what phase she is in in her cycle. With your fingers, gently circle the cervix, where there are subtle energies that can be released through this touch. Usually women will not specifically feel this touch on the cervix.

2. **Fisting:** In some women it is possible at this point to very gently insert the entire hand into the yoni. This requires a great deal of trust and relaxation. If this is not possible, insert as many fingers as possible very, very slowly into the yoni. During this time, the receiving woman should take deep breaths to allow her to build up a lot of *ching chi.*

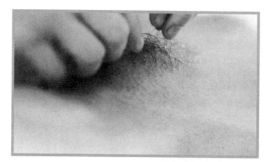

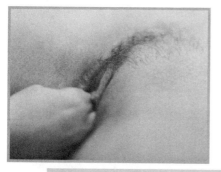 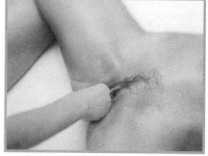

Phase 8: The Finale—Calming the Energy and Closing the Gates

3. **Quiet:** Remain still and let your fingers or hand rest in the yoni. Do not move at all, but remain very aware. After that, in slow motion, pull out your fingers or hand.

4. **Distributing energy:** Distribute the energy by stroking in the direction of the legs, abdomen, head, and arms.

5. **Close the gates:** Place your hands on the anus and yoni and mentally close the gates.

6. **The Big Draw:** The receiving woman takes a deep breath and tenses her whole body: fists, feet, legs, arms, abdomen, shoulders, and face. Holding her breath, she maintains this tension for as long as possible before letting go and relaxing (for a fuller description, see page 85).

7. Now cover your partner with a cloth and do not touch her. In this way, she can concentrate fully on herself and on the movement of energy in her body. With or without the Big Draw, it is very important that the woman is left alone with herself for a while now. If she were to get up immediately after this intense experience, she could miss the very valuable after-feelings. The giver can be present during this time but should not interfere physically or energetically in the system of the partner. Simply being there is enough.

8. In the after-feeling phase, all the experiences that were awakened dur-

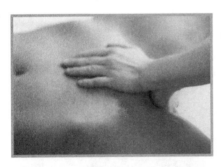
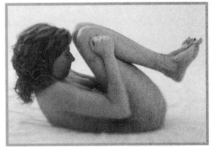
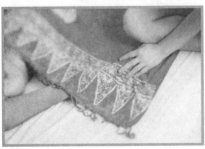
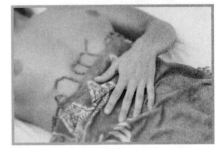

Phase 8

ing the yoni massage can unfold. Body and psyche process the released information and transform it into consciousness. Many women report trancelike conditions, intense feelings, prickling sensations in the body, and perception of colors or smells.

℘ *Phase 9: Saying Farewell*

The ninth and last phase is what I call "farewell." In this phase, the shared experience between the giver and the receiver is rounded and closed. This is the time to say or ask about anything that needs to be resolved, and perhaps to hear the receiving woman talk briefly about her experience (if she wishes to). After this, the yoni massage is finished, and both parties can leave the space well grounded and with clarity. This is an important phase for many women, since after such intense shared experiences they tend to remain linked to one another. In our practice, however, we are dealing with a content-oriented collaboration that needs to have a clearly defined end. Of course, this doesn't mean that a yoni massage shouldn't be carried out within a romantic relationship, but even these should have some kind of clearly defined end, to allow the partners to return to the normal give-and-take of their relationship.

Namaste—I greet the godly in you.

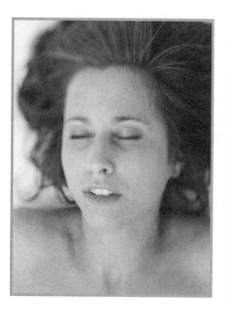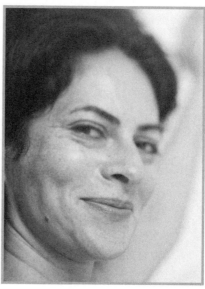

Phase 9: Saying Farewell

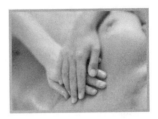

CONCLUDING THOUGHTS

Those who begin to encounter their sexuality in a conscious way never walk the path for themselves alone. We create waves that will gradually affect others as well, spreading the experience of healing and the understanding of ourselves and our desires.

Your own healing will change you. You will teach your children differently and will explain their sexuality to them in a more conscious, knowledgeable, and understandable way, allowing the next generation to be free of some of the misconceptions that have limited us. For this I thank all those people who have had the courage to deal with their sexuality in a healing way. And we will need this courage, since our society continues to be far from the point of recognizing people who have made a conscious decision in favor of a healthier sexuality and who are working toward that end. In this regard, we are all pioneers and can all follow one guiding principle: it is about love!

Experience Reports

Earth

In this night she was ready
And saw
And was earth
Earth in her body, in her veins
In all pores
Never felt so intensively
Full of tenderness and power
And called to herself the words of the
mother:

Life   love   strength

And was forever filled with this call
Did, was ready,
For the volcano in her belly to erupt—
Finally
Unending strength
Strength from earth

Let walls glide softly around the small body
You are complete

Let hands glide softly around the small body
You are welcome

Welcome on earth.

—ANTONIA ALARIS

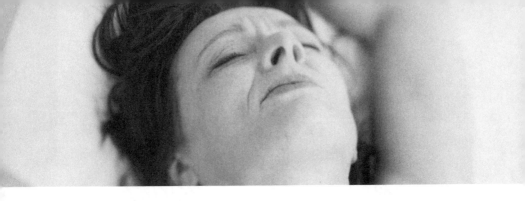

To reflect the experiences of women as authentically as possible, I interviewed a number of them directly after their yoni massages. These interviews are recorded here verbatim, although I have left out certain passages that would be of little interest to readers or that would be too intimate for the woman in question for publication. Sometimes I also rephrased some statements for better readability.

Most of these women come from my circle of friends and acquaintances or were guests at AnandaWave. They are women who have been dealing intensively with their sexuality for some time. I thank the women who took part in these interviews with all my heart, including those whose interviews I did not include here. These examples offer an insight into the variety of experiences that women can have during a yoni massage. The names were changed to protect the identity of the women in question.

YONI MASSAGE WITH CARMEN

Carmen: That was great! I'm still a little dazed [laughs]. I have to drink something. That was fantastic. I haven't had such great sensations in a long time. Never, actually.

Michaela: Does that include the touching of the yoni area too?

Carmen: Especially there. Of course, that was also a main goal of mine. Everything else was totally great to get down, but the yoni massage was really good. I mean, now we don't need men anymore, do we? [Both laugh.] They could never do this. Great. I don't have this kind of experience with a man.

Michaela: Does that mean that when you sleep with a man, your feelings are not this good?

Carmen: No, it's good, but just not like this was. I have nice feelings, but they don't reach the same spots that you did . . .

Michaela: What were those spots?

Carmen: Well, I felt everything pretty deeply. I mean, I don't know what exactly you did there. That's one thing I meant to ask you: what exactly did you do with your hands? It felt so full.

Michaela: I was inside you, with two, three, sometimes even four fingers.

Carmen: Great! [Both laugh out loud.]

Michaela: I can't do that with every woman.

Carmen: No? Why not?

Michaela: Well, with many women, all that fits is one finger.

Carmen: You mean because of space?

Michaela: Yes. And sometimes they close up and are too tight. That wasn't the case with you at all—you could even open up further. You have space. A lot of space.

Carmen: What would you say about the problems that I told you about earlier?

Michaela: You mean that you can't reach orgasm?

Carmen: I have to practice a bit, no?

Michaela: Yes. I get the sense that you are not in touch with your clitoris.

Carmen: That's true, I'm not. I don't think about it a great deal.

Michaela: Well, many women find it easiest to reach orgasm via their clitoris, so it's worth getting to know it better.

Carmen: Hmm. But I have no reactions from my clitoris at all.

Michaela: For many women, the opposite is the case. They often don't feel a whole lot from my entering their yoni and often show their reactions only via the clitoris.

Carmen: I had much more intensive reactions when you were inside my yoni.

Michaela: That's true, I noticed that too. Especially in rather unusual spots, even far down. How was that for you when I turned my fingers around and reach further down?

Carmen: That's exactly what I liked, the fact that it was so varied and kept changing. I found myself thinking: wow, what's that? There is a great space inside where one can play. Kind of like I had that sensation before but didn't know how or what or where. And there were things that I didn't know at all, because I don't touch myself in that way.

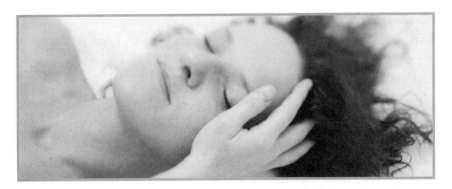

Michaela: Well, it would be rather difficult to do that on yourself.

Carmen: That's right, I would really have to contort myself. But what do I do now that I know that I am more receptive to stimulation inside than outside? That doesn't work so well for me, because I don't get so much from my clitoris.

Michaela: You will definitely need to work on building up contact with your clitoris.

Carmen: You mean I have to really practice that?

Michaela: I would say yes, that's how women collect their experiences. When I think of myself, I began playing with my clitoris and kept trying until it worked at one point.

Carmen: Well, I have played with it, but I don't feel anything while doing it and eventually didn't enjoy it anymore. Or there were only brief nice moments that surprised me, but then my head switched back to "not interested."

Michaela: Do you fantasize when you have sex?

Carmen: No, I don't really think of anything. If I do, it's only a brief thought, but I can't get into it, it switches on and off.

Michaela: But aren't there any images or scenes from television that you find erotic?

Carmen: Well yes, there are some things.

Michaela: It makes sense to use everything that can help you in any way.

Carmen: I have to somehow be able to make the leap to get into that. I already have problems expressing myself during sex or even making a noise. It's already a lot that I am at least breathing now; normally I hold my breath. I think my biggest problem is that I don't want to lose control, so as not to lose anything. I have to work on reducing that.

Michaela: That's true, especially because your body is there—it hasn't closed up.

Carmen: No?

Michaela: No—I thought your yoni was very open. I see that you are too much in your head, but there are others who have bigger problems and are still able to orgasm.

Carmen: Really? Why not me? Even though I always get the feeling that I am so close.

Michaela: Yes, you were very close.

Carmen: Why am I like this? Does it have to be this way? I'm really confused—you read so many different things describing orgasm in the most fantastic ways. But I don't feel like I am experiencing anything like an explosion. It's true there are sensations that are not exactly everyday, it is pleasant and great and I think I could spend hours lying there enjoying myself. But I don't know what has to happen. Perhaps I am trying too hard to understand this.

Michaela: There are many maybes, and I think anything I would say at this point will only leave you thinking about it more. So the only thing I will say is play around with it. Buy some oil and simply keep trying. Usually, an orgasm comes when we expect it least. It is important not to want an orgasm too much, it will come by itself when the time is right. I also think that you have never masturbated, which means that you have never built up your own contact with your yoni. The only contact you have is with the inside of it when you have sex with a man and that's why that works better for you; that's where you draw your experience from. This experience is missing for your clitoris.

Carmen: That's right, exactly right. And of course most men don't spend a lot of time making this nice for you also from the outside. But now I want to know what I like where, and how I can get there by myself.

Michaela: Well, you are in the process of doing just that. Do you want to tell me more about what you experienced during the yoni massage?

Carmen: Well, for the first time I felt that I had different parts in my yoni that had different reactions. And then I used my pelvis, which I completely forgot at the beginning. At some point I just began feeling it, and thought, "Oh right, that somehow is part of you too—I should use it."

Michaela: Yes, that definitely supports the massage.

Carmen: I was surprised what different spots there are, especially because I always look for the G-spot within me but can never seem to find it.

Michaela: Did you have the ability to feel it during the massage?

Carmen: I'm not sure. There were a number of points in this that I enjoyed. Especially the simultaneous, outside and inside, I liked that. I noticed that.

Michaela: So also including the clitoris?

Carmen: Yes, but further down actually, more near the entrance. I liked that better. On the clitoris I felt rather little, I have to say. But thank God you always kept a finger inside me. That was good, because I think that otherwise not as much would have happened.

Michaela: At the very end, I spent some time massaging only the clitoris . . .

Carmen: Yes, I liked that too. That was very nice and became more pleasant toward the end, more intense.

Michaela: There you have it.

Carmen: I thought, there is something there, that shouldn't simply be ignored the way I do it all the time. But it took a long time before there was any feeling there.

Michaela: Well, the clitoris is simply still asleep, in a deep sleep.

Carmen: I can't believe it! Where everything else is awake inside me.

Michaela: It's because you don't touch it! I mean . . .

Carmen: Yes, but what if it doesn't wake up?

Michaela: It will.

Carmen: Are you sure?

Michaela: Yes, I'm sure of it.

Carmen: Well, then it will be all right, then I don't have anything too bad ahead of me. You were very deep inside my yoni, right?

Michaela: I turned my hands around and massaged especially your uterus.

Carmen: That was very pleasant.

Michaela: Yes, I always massage the uterus. In some women I can hardly reach it, but that wasn't a problem with you. It is not so smooth inside you, there are valleys and hills, which is very interesting. Every once in a while I found a little cave into which I could dig.

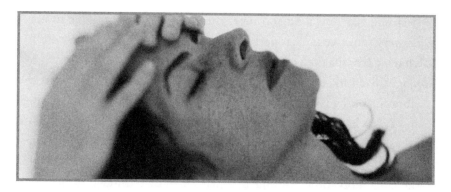

Carmen: Really? I will have to look for myself what is going on in there. I can't believe what you are telling me about the great things I have inside me.

Michaela: It is definitely very exciting inside your yoni. There is a lot to discover.

Carmen: Everything that was new and that I discovered in emotions was great. There was nothing negative in it—nothing at all. And then I even found my own rhythm in a way, which I usually find difficult to do.

Michaela: Well then, on to new shores. Thank you for this conversation.

YONI MASSAGE WITH SONJA

Michaela: How do you feel?

Sonja: Great. It was very nice. My feeling was so deep; I didn't think I would be able to relax so completely.

Michaela: Do you know yourself to be different, that you are not usually able to relax as much?

Sonja: No, I can usually let go quite well, but I thought that with you . . . the situation might be a bit more difficult. But I enjoyed it a lot.

Michaela: Have you had many yoni massages?

Sonja: Not many. Perhaps about eight of them.

Michaela: How was the massage for you on the whole? What were your feelings about the massage as a whole, or was there something in particular that you noticed about it? We can also talk about the massage step by step.

Sonja: I thought the massage was absolutely great, especially that you touched me a little more firmly at times. Only at the front of the stomach, that was a bit too firm. But that is perhaps unique to me, I am very sensitive in that part of my body, that is my intimate area.

Michaela: No, that's the case with many women.

Sonja: What I liked about the yoni massage right from the start was the vibrating of the yoni during the chakra balancing. You only did it once, and I also know it's been done three times. I once had a really intense experience with that, in which I could feel that channel and the different chakras very intensively. I also liked how much time you took for the labia, both inner and outer. I needed to be reminded of how nice it is when they get that much attention. Now I feel that they are really thick and well circulated. It feels as if they are flowering, and I liked that a lot. I especially liked the way you applied pressure on the inner labia, directed toward the inside; that touched me very deeply.

Michaela: How did this depth feel for you?

Sonja: By deep I mean that I felt how the internal organs were being stimulated. How the energy was being channeled toward the inside, creating a feeling that went below the surface. I don't know how else to put it.

Michaela: Let's continue step by step. How was the stimulation of the clitoris for you?

Sonja: That was almost too much.

Michaela: I almost thought as much. But what exactly was it about that? Was it too firm?

Sonja: No, I don't know whether you know this, but I had a similar feeling at the beginning when you stroked the front of my body with feathers. I get a prickling sensation in my mouth that I almost can't stand.

Michaela: In your mouth?

Sonja: Yes [laughs]. That is not only about the clitoris. You also couldn't have continued with the feathers, otherwise I would have jumped up. The feeling is intensely arousing, but there is something where it crosses over and becomes too much. With the clitoris, it was at that limit.

Michaela: Perhaps it was too light? It is possible that I touched you too lightly and should have applied more pressure.

Sonja: No, the point is not that anything was wrong or that it needed this or that. Everything was right, and I would have told you if it had become too much. I know this and find it interesting that it starts in the mouth—very strange. The whole feeling starts at the surface of the gums, that's where I notice it the most. Do you know this?

Michaela: In the yoni I only know that state of overstimulation, if something was too firm and arousal is mixed with pain.

Sonja: For me it doesn't have to be firm. A gentle touch is enough.

Michaela: Very interesting. And then I entered your yoni and massaged it intensively from the inside.

Sonja: That was simply very pleasant.

Michaela: Was there anything that felt funny or different in that?

Sonja: When you were inside me with your fingers I really liked feeling the entrance of the yoni in that way. That made the massage very holistic. Then I was very surprised to suddenly have experienced such an orgasm wave. I didn't expect that.

Michaela: Was it a real orgasm or just a wave?

Sonja: It was a real orgasm, but a very gentle one. Very pleasant. Nothing ecstatic or explosive, but more a letting go.

Michaela: At some point, I massaged both your G-spot inside and your clitoris outside. How did the stimulation of your clitoris feel then? Did you again experience the prickling sensation in your mouth?

Sonja: No, that was very, very nice.

Michaela: The feeling is probably distributed better when the yoni is stimulated simultaneously.

Sonja: I don't know exactly why. Before, when you massaged only the clitoris, I thought you could make a break in between, to simply hold the clitoris for a while. To simply hold the energy a few times to allow it to go even deeper.

Michaela: I would be really angry if someone started, then stopped, started, then stopped. [Laughter.] How different we women are. Did you notice that I also massaged your cervix?

Sonja: Not directly.

Michaela: Your uterus is very far to the front; it has a relatively strong bend to the front.

Sonja: My gynecologist noted the same. I was positively surprised when she simply noted "there is nothing funny about it, the uterus is simply the way it is, it has a bend," in contrast to what the other doctors always tell us.

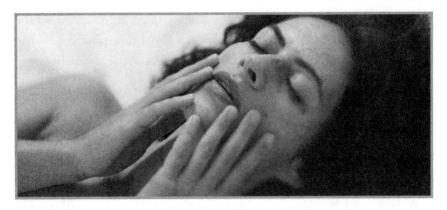

Michaela: It's the typical category thinking. Anything that doesn't correspond to the norm is automatically not normal and thus ill.

Sonja: About the whole massage, I can simply say again how much I enjoyed it to be touched so lovingly and intensely for such a long time. That is a really big gift. I also really noted that you enjoyed giving the massage, and that made it all the better.

Michaela: I would also be interested in hearing how you are experiencing your sexuality in general. How do you live it? What have you experienced so far? A little bit about your sexual history.

Sonja: Sex is the part of my life that is the least complicated. That has always been the case for me.

Michaela: Right from the beginning, including the first time?

Sonja: Right from the beginning. I am lucky in that way. Don't ask me why, but it was always normal for me. I always thought that was the case for everyone until I learned that for most people it's not this way. That is also one reason why I am on this tantric path. I have completely godly experiences with it. I was always lucky in my sexuality, even during pregnancy.

Michaela: So that the men always fit?

Sonja: Yes [laughs], the men always fit, too. Except sometimes in long-term relationships, then I sometimes have a problem that the man has problems and no longer can or wants to. At one time, a man had a history of abuse, which he had realized, and after which sex was difficult for him. Another man had prostate problems for which he had to take medication and then was unable to have sex.

Michaela: What do you do when you are in a relationship and the man is not able to perform sexually?

Sonja: To be honest, after a long back and forth and a lot of pain, we eventually separated. And after the separation I lived my freedom, experimented a lot. When I began to meditate, my sexuality changed even more. It became a prayer, especially with men who also meditated. That is simply the most spiritual experience I have had to date. But unfortunately there are not many such men [laughs]. I have been without sex for a couple of months now.

Michaela: And how do you deal with sexuality during such times? Do you masturbate a lot then, or do you say, okay, I don't need this?

Sonja: No, I need it. I can pleasure myself, but would like to have a man again.

Michaela: Who wouldn't? [Laughs.] How was your sexuality during pregnancy?

Sonja: During my pregnancy I had a great time with sex. Only the last couple of months were difficult, since it is a bit strange when the child is larger and there is penetration—the child is really pushed then. Otherwise sexuality was an area in which I had no problems at all.

Michaela: And no bad experiences? It's so rare, that's why I am asking.

Sonja: For me, it was always normal. I just always had very clear limits when it came to sex. Of course, every once in a while I had a date where I thought, what kind of guy is this? But it never went past a certain limit. My parents are also pretty free on this topic.

Michaela: Thank you for this conversation.

YONI MASSAGE WITH ANNA

Michaela: You are not feeling so well and have a cold—was the massage nonetheless good for you?

Anna: Yes it was. I was really able to let go during it. And the yoni massage was a real journey. By the end, during the second part, I noticed that I wanted to fulfill certain expectations, for example to give feedback through movements or noises, et cetera. I know that from sex too. Of course I know that you don't have these expectations, but still I couldn't help feel them. And then I also noticed, wow, how deep-seated that is, and how little I am able to simply lie there. At the beginning of the massage that was no problem at all, but when it took an arousing direction, I very quickly felt an expectation to show a reaction. I noticed how I judged myself: "Hey, you are simply lying there, stiff as a board, not doing anything."

Michaela: Yes, these feelings have very deep roots. That is the case for many women, even when they are in the middle of experiencing arousal. I know that from my own experience as well, to feel the need to add to the natural reaction. It makes no sense, but is difficult to fight in the moment.

Anna: Yes, it's simply there and there is nothing I could do against it. I always note then that I quickly become too tense. For a while there is a natural need to move and to express my feelings, but then I realize that I am also working myself into it and remain in a tension that doesn't allow for relaxation.

Michaela: Where the movement is no longer smooth, but conscious and rigid?

Anna: It becomes more and more conscious. And then comes this longing for orgasm. Where you want it so much and then it doesn't work at all. Where it is no longer possible to relax and you become increasingly tense, looking for resolution, but feeling blocked. I don't know what that is.

Michaela: What and how do you think in moments like those? What are your mental loops?

Anna: Well, if it's about orgasm, then I become impatient and think the whole time along the lines of "I hope this doesn't take too long." In that way, I put pressure on myself and am worried to be taking too long. But that wasn't the case just now. It was good that you said at the beginning that it is not about reaching orgasm, but about a journey, about feeling and discovery. That was very nice, and I reminded myself of that and gave myself over to simply feeling.

Michaela: You just said that you sometimes think "I hope this doesn't take too long." Have you experienced orgasms when you were intimate with men?

Anna: I have always been close, always had a feeling of being almost there.

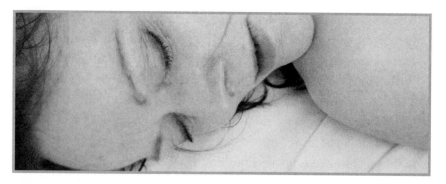

I think I only had an actual orgasm twice, more or less by accident, completely unexpected.

Michaela: Always in moments where you probably least expected it.

Anna: Exactly.

Michaela: That's so crazy, I wish one could trick oneself past that in some way.

Anna: I wish that too.

Michaela: But unfortunately we are clever and stupid at the same time. And how was it with the yoni massage? What did you like, what was not so pleasant? How was your journey and what happened to you during it?

Anna: Well, what I really liked was the very slow approach—I knew where it was going, but you very gently approached the whole area. I really liked that. And the warmth and pressure on the yoni was incredible, that really went through my body. I also noticed that you massaged the vaginal opening pretty firmly at the beginning and immediately noted that hurts, that feels sore. That was my old feeling again. I didn't say anything about that to you, perhaps also because I didn't think of it. The entire first exploration was rather tense for me.

Michaela: The one where I was inside you for a long time?

Anna: Yes, that wasn't really nice.

Michaela: What exactly was it that didn't feel really good? Was it too dry and uncomfortable for that reason?

Anna: No, I'm never too dry, that's the crazy thing. I am always totally wet, but there is a soreness there that I find difficult to explain. I notice that I am tense and very careful. Okay, if it had been unbearable, of course I would have said something, but in this case, I only observed it and tried to remember. That feeling only went away when you switched to the last position. I don't know, were you inside me with your thumb then? That was really great, and I was able to relax completely.

Michaela: Your yoni has a slight downward bend, and when I enter it with my thumb, it more closely mirrors the direction of your yoni. In this way, I could move without pushing up against it.

Anna: Everything that involves pushing against the wall is unpleasant for me. That is a stimulation that I find disturbing. No matter how much you stimulate the clitoris, it really distracts me, and I am no longer able to enjoy anything. Of course that's always difficult to communicate during sex, and today I noticed that I only thought of saying something when you had found the nice position and then wanted to return. It was only then that I noticed, no, I don't want that. Otherwise I was thinking, okay, this is a journey of discovery, that's part of it, that is what it is like in my yoni. That frustrated me a lot.

Michaela: That you are unable to define your limits?

Anna: That too of course, but also that I am so complicated. That I am so sensitive to pain and pressure and have to direct things so much. Of course my partners also felt limited, because I was always saying like this, not like that, not yet, slow, et cetera . . . I am always directing and they cannot just go for it. That is of course annoying for them and difficult for me.

Michaela: When you sleep with someone, do you have this soreness automatically from the beginning?

Anna: No, it varies. It also has to do with the body of the partner. The

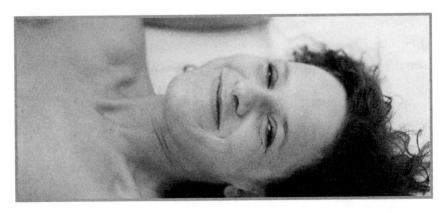

smaller and more pointed the penis, the better. With a little cute one it's okay. It can also be long—as long as it is thin. [Laughter.] Decisive is the openness, how open I can be in the moment. There are situations, though they are very rare, where it simple slides in and later I hardly have any problems at all. But very often it is that I don't notice anything while we are actually doing it, but the next day I am sore and have to walk with my legs apart. It feels so sore that even the underwear feels like it is rubbing. That is very frustrating.

Michaela: It really does seem to have something to do with openness, and in fact I too know moments like those you describe. If the encounter isn't right nothing works, everything hurts, but the next time everything can be all right again. Which to me suggests that the problem does not lie in the yoni.

Anna: You probably didn't notice any limits inside me, or did you?

Michaela: When I had two fingers inside you, I did notice that. I was briefly unsure, which is rare for me. Especially because you were very wet and nothing felt uneven or hard, so I really thought that it felt completely soft, great, and easy for you.

Anna: Would it have been better for you if I had said something?

Michaela: Of course, I would have gone more slowly then, or stopped in between, to make sure that everything was all right for you.

Anna: Somehow the thought didn't even cross my mind. I somehow thought, this is the massage, and this is what you do. But, of course, that is stupid. I could have said something.

Michaela: Especially because that was a long part of the massage. But it is what it is, so this is part of it too then.

Anna: Yes, for me it is another experience that shows that I am not good at setting limits. And yet sometimes I think how easy it all could be.

Michaela: There is often information that is rooted so deep in our bodies that we at first don't have a chance to control it directly. It happens gradually, as we become more aware of it. Let us walk through the yoni massage step by step. How was it with the labia, the inner and outer?

Anna: Actually, already then I felt the soreness. Around the outside was really beautiful, I think that was before you touched the labia. With the labia it was already too strong. The sensitivity is really enormous. I have it in my everyday life too, when I would love to walk around naked, feeling that even wearing pants is too much. And yet at the same time I was thinking to myself that it was not about enjoyment but discovery.

Michaela: Perhaps I should have been more clear at the beginning that limits are limits and that discovery can also be related to enjoyment.

Anna: Yes, perhaps that would have been good. In sex, of course, it is very clear that it is about pleasure, and there I by now say stop when I find it uncomfortable. But I guess I saw this massage from a different angle.

Michaela: I can understand your thoughts behind that; it's something that could happen to me too. How was it when I touched your clitoris?

Anna: That was simply beautiful. The way you touched it too was simply wonderful. In those moments I was able to relax completely.

Michaela: And when I was outside you with both fingers, during the tapping?

Anna: Oh, that was great too. You did that near the beginning, yum. Even before that you stroked the clitoris and entered the yoni with a very delicate pressure, I also really liked that. There was no resistance there at all, and you moved in a really nice way. For me, that was probably the best part, being so still inside me and moving back and forth gently. Nothing spectacular perhaps, but you did it a lot, simply being inside and focusing on the clitoris.

Michaela: How was the end phase for you where I did that for a very long time?

Anna: I was able to completely enjoy it, and it was then that I began to trust the situation more. Of course, I still had the comments in my head that I should move more, should give you feedback, should not simply lie there—that whole garbage. But then I told myself, no, you know that, just lie there and enjoy simply lying there. For me, that was a very deep moment. There was a very deep wave of enjoyment there, but it did not last long; then came the next quality. I thought it was interesting that it kept changing. You cannot simply hold on to the pleasure. You can enjoy it, only to let go of it again. Then you can be surprised by what comes next. I noticed very positively that it was worthwhile letting go, rather than trying to hold on to it. I like doing that but often tense up in the process. Then I had a few moments of "How much time do we still have, this seems to have gone on so long already,

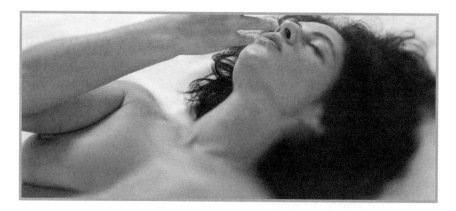

will I have an orgasm or not," which took up a lot of my attention.

Michaela: I also noticed that you were concerned about time.

Anna: It was nice for me to see that you simply stayed with it. That felt good. Then I was disappointed for a very short moment when I noted that you were closing the gates. By the way, as a gesture it was really beautiful when you really closed the labia. I thought that was a very nice gesture, very loving and respectful. Respecting the opening.

Michaela: And at the end you were in a nice wave?

Anna: Yes, and it kept getting stronger. For me, the massage could have continued for longer, also because I was curious whether I would have been able to have an orgasm in these waves of highs and lows. Also with you, because although I know you, I don't know you that well. And finally, perhaps something would have been possible in this situation that wouldn't be possible otherwise. There was a curiosity there, coupled with a knowledge that we had probably already spent three hours.

Michaela: I think it would be good for you to receive these yoni massages more frequently, to learn to better cope with certain patterns, for example to say stop. To say that you would like to go in this direction, because you like that better. And to find out more about what you enjoy. Through this you can begin to build up trust in your own opening. You can learn to trust yourself, which I think is what this is about with you.

Anna: The crazy thing is that I have this longing for sex, for this feeling of having something inside me. I love that feeling and miss it. It's not as if I don't want something inside me. There is this crazy contradiction going on inside me.

Michaela: I'm sure that contradiction is driving you crazy. Were you able to talk about it in your relationships?

Anna: Yes, I usually tried to talk about it, but I also noted that it was a bit of a burden. While most partners were open about it, they didn't know what to do with it. And of course I ask myself what messages I was sending during the communication. I say that I am sensitive and not sure myself how to handle it. But men are very quickly in a role then: how do I fix that? And they don't know the answer.

Michaela: I would imagine that in this situation they encounter their own insecurities, with their own doubts about their abilities. I can understand that.

Anna: Yes, I think it's often frustrating for them because they feel as if they are not doing it right.

Michaela: And they don't have a success experience, which I think is very important to men when it comes to sex. Not only with men, incidentally. By the way, how was your relationship with your parents when it came to sex? Was this topic discussed, or was it rather taboo?

Anna: It was a catastrophe. I think that's where all of this started. My parents were very religious, they are anthroposophist, 180 percent, and were not very open about physical things. They were naturalists, and we were often nude, in terms of swimming on holiday, or running around the house as children. But everything related to sensuality, lust, and sexuality was taboo.

Michaela: So the topic simply didn't exist?

Anna: Kissing, cuddling, and being tender was simply not possible for my mother; there were too many of us. She was completely overwhelmed with the household and all the children. I was the fourth, but there were some more that followed after me, and I always felt like I wasn't getting quite enough. Then I had a boyfriend, and that was a real cuddling relationship. That's where I made up for everything that I didn't get from my parents; it was a wonderful sense of fulfillment. But my parents didn't like this at all. When we went into a room to cuddle and my little siblings came in, my mother would always get them, she was worried that they would see that the two of us were physically close. And she said that quite openly: walking hand in hand on the street was a bad example to set for the little ones. I deeply absorbed that it

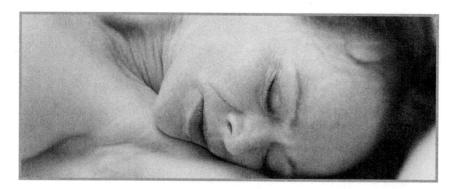

was something bad, and it took a long time until I created a different picture.

Michaela: Yes, that can take an eternity. In fact, I think it's a lifelong process.

Anna: It was very difficult for me.

Michaela: I'm sure it wasn't much different for your siblings than it was for you.

Anna: No, but they had different ways of dealing with it. All the girls are very much tomboys. I am the only one who is so feminine. I was always the crybaby too, very fragile as a child, and I often had the feeling that I carried the sensitive side for all of them. It was always a little rough at home, loving and nice to one another, not fighting, but rough in the demeanor. I always felt that my nature left me a little apart from everyone else.

Michaela: And how was your first period?

Anna: It was a catastrophe. Everything that had to do with sexuality went wrong. Sex ed was a very delicate thing, taboo times ten. I asked my older sister what sex was since everyone in class was talking about it, but she only said ask Mom. Then I asked my mother, and her reaction was: oh no, what do we do now. Then she got the four older ones together and sat us down in the living room. Then my father began talking about love. "It can be very nice, for example for two people to go for a walk, or for a boy to invite a girl to the movies." And so on, even though I only wanted to know how it works. But he stuck with his story: that they get to know each other better, get married, and then at some point have children. "And when do you know that a child is coming?" I asked my mother that question at some later point in

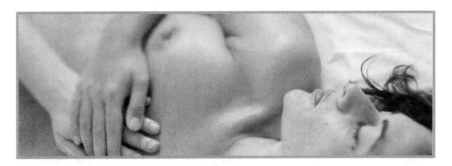

time. It was a serious question, and her response was, "There comes the archangel." And that was what I learned about sex.

My first period came when we were on a class trip, and it was horrible. I was very premenstrual, had mood swings and felt like crying, and all the people from my class had first a pillow fight and then an orange fight. They all had their fun and I was simply crying. I had painful abdominal cramps and felt terrible, the way it goes when someone can't join the fun. And of course, that's when everyone turns on you. All of a sudden I had all the smashed-up oranges in my bed. "All against Anna," and bam. Nobody noticed that I was feeling bad; in their eyes I was simply staying outside of the fun. That left a deep mark on me, this connection of menstruation and feeling bad, the pain and feeling like an outcast. It keeps coming up when I menstruate.

My mother never understood any of this. I would come home from school because the pain was so bad that I couldn't walk anymore, and her comment was only, "Now again you come home so early, you could at least have stayed for gym class. I always went to gym class, even when I had my period." She only reprimanded me, but she didn't understand how terrible the pain was. Sometimes I had the worst cramps for days on end, couldn't go to school, really couldn't, threw up and had nightmares, and she would still say I should go to school. At some point I yelled at her, "You are a terrible mother," and shut the door in her face, because I was so exhausted. She had no understanding, zero, and I really feel that something broke at that point in our relationship.

Michaela: My goodness. That is why it is so important that we make progress on this topic of sexuality, so that the next generation can breathe a little easier. Thank you for this conversation.

The Origin and History of Yoni Massage

Yoni massage as I teach it has amusing origins. In 1982 Joseph Kramer developed Taoist Erotic Massage—a spiritual-erotic bodywork that focused primarily on breathing and massage techniques. He himself spent years studying the teachings of Taoism and familiarized himself with the body's entire meridian system. From the point of view of Taoist sexual teachings, arousal and sexual energy circulate in the body. "Taoist massage" and conscious breathing support and intensify this circulation of energy. Since Kramer himself is gay, an important part of the massage was the massage of the lingam, the male genitals. Unique about this massage was that men did not ejaculate but experienced the circulation of energy throughout their whole body. This was completely new for many of the people that Joseph taught in San Francisco. Because of the spread of AIDS in the 1980s, men were even more ready to have such erotic experiences, and in this way learned the joy and advantages of sexuality without ejaculation.

Joseph made a few audiotapes for teaching materials that he titled "Ecstatic Sex" and "Healthy Sex." Annie Sprinkle listened to these tapes in 1986 and immediately fell in love with his voice. Annie had been a prostitute and artist since she was eighteen and referred to herself as a sexual healer. At the time, she was editor of *Penthouse* magazine and was preparing an issue that dealt with spirituality and spiritual sex. From the audiotapes it quickly became apparent that Joseph knew a lot about sexuality, so she called him and invited him to an interview for the magazine. The two met in New York for the interview.

Following this, Annie attended a breathing course with Joseph that he called "Tantric Rebirthing." She was the only woman among forty gay men. For three hours the group breathed together and Annie experienced, fully clothed, her first great "energy orgasm," stretching from her head to her hands and into her toes. In this, she had a very emotional, spiritual, liberating physical experience. From that day onward, she wanted to learn from Joseph everything he could teach her.

Joseph had never before met someone who had as much to say about sexuality as he did, and who talked about it as much. He was surprised and fell in love, describing it as a kind of trance. Annie loved Joseph in the same way, and things were wonderful from the start. A gay man and a woman with changing sexual orientations became friends and lovers who complemented each other on many levels.

Then the ideas began to flow. Annie and Joseph continuously created new images related to sex. Annie taught and acted in theater, did her shows, and began to develop her own performances. Joseph traveled the United States and Europe, especially Germany, and taught "erotic touch" for homosexual men. Their paths continued to cross, and they met in Hamburg, Amsterdam, Los Angeles, San Francisco, New York, and New Orleans. Their encounters were always wonderful, and both felt a strong connection to the other. Annie wanted to experience as a woman the erotic massages that Joseph taught for men. She wanted Joseph to massage her.

He was a professional masseur but had never before given an erotic genital massage to a woman. He asked her to help him and let her guide him. Through her breathing, Annie quickly entered an erotic trance, from which she said that the two would have to work together to develop this massage for women.

In 1993 they worked together to develop the first steps of yoni massage and the names for the individual phases that continue to be used today. Annie taught Joseph a lot about female anatomy, and together they learned and evaluated what he had done with her during the massage. Shortly thereafter they taught a seminar called "Cosmic Orgasm Awareness Week" to forty men and women in a retreat center in northern California.

The focus of the yoni massage lies on the massage rather than on sex. The primary focus is touch. As an experienced masseur, Joseph knew that the entire body awakens when it is massaged and touched. This experience is what Joseph and Annie applied to the massage in the female genital area. What was important for the awakening process was that the receiving woman breathed consciously, since breathing brings attention to the body. This is the origin of yoni massage.

The sexual coach, educator, and researcher K. Ruby mentioned above was one participant in this first "Cosmic Orgasm Awareness Week" and there encountered a yoni massage, which up to that point had been practiced more like a male genital massage. Later, Ruby herself taught these workshops, along with Chester Mainard, one of the teachers from Joseph Kramer's San Francisco–based Body Electric School. During this period, K. Ruby refined the yoni massage to what it is today, with its phases, steps, and framework more attuned to the needs of women. She and Chester Mainard added depth to the yoni massage.

The Body Electric School brought this massage to Germany, where I experienced it in 1995 as part of a tantric ritual and have now finally, after years of collecting experiences, written the first book ever on this topic.

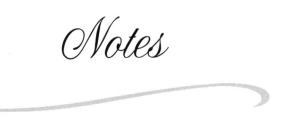

Notes

CHAPTER 1. FEMALE SEXUALITY

1. Sabine zur Nieden, *Weibliche Ejakulation* [Female Ejaculation] (Giessen, Germany: Psychosocial Publishers, 2004), 23.

2. Jane Patterson et al., *Frauenkörper neu gesehen* [Female Bodies in a New Light] (Berlin: Orlanda Frauenverlag, 1997), 38.

3. Barbara G. Walker, *Das geheime Wissen der Frauen* [The Secret Knowledge of Women] (Uhlstädt-Kirchhasel, Germany: Arun Publishers, 2003), 549. Originally published in English as *The Woman's Encyclopedia of Myths and Secrets.*

4. Carlos Castaneda, *Tensegrity: Die magischen Bewegungen der Zauberer* [Tensegrity: The Magic Movements of Magicians] (Frankfurt: Fischer Publishers, 1998), 76.

5. Interview with Günter Schmale, M.D., a general practitioner and pharmacist in Cologne, Germany, who focuses on acupuncture and homeopathy and is a user of the "Tzentimeter" method.

6. Source: *Connection Special,* VI/04.

7. Interview with Günter Schmale, M.D.

8. Natalie Angier, *Frau: Eine intime Geographie des weiblichen Körpers* [Woman: An Intimate Geography of the Female Body] (Munich: Goldmann Publishers, 2002), 33–34. Originally published in English as *Woman: An Intimate Geography.*

9. Interview with Günter Schmale, M.D.

10. Christiane Northtrup, M.D., *Frauenkörper, Frauenweisheit: Wie Frauen ihre ursprüngliche Fähigkeit zur Selbstheilung wiederentdecken können* [Women's

Bodies, Women's Wisdom: How Women Can Rediscover Their Original Self-Healing Abilities] (Munich: Zabert Sanmann Publishers, 2003), 226. Originally published in English as *Women's Bodies, Women's Wisdom: Creating Physical and Emotional Health and Healing*.

11. Zur Nieden, *Weibliche Ejakulation*, 18.

12. Ibid.

13. Ibid.

14. Ibid., 24.

15. Ibid.

16. Ibid., 25.

17. Ibid., 31.

18. Eva Rudy Jansen, *Die Bildersprache des Hinduismus: Göttinnen und Götter, Erscheinungsformen und Bedeutungen* [The Language of Images in Hinduism: Gods and Goddesses, Apparations and Their Meanings] (Publisher NA: 1993), 135. Published in English as *The Book of Hindu Imagery: The Gods and Their Symbols*.

19. Northrup, *Frauenkörper, Frauenweisheit*, 146.

20. Nik Douglas and Penny Slinger, *Das grosse Buch des Tantra: Sexuelle Geheimnisse und die Alchemie der Ekstase* [The Big Book of Tantra: Sexual Secrets and the Alchemy of Ecstasy] (Munich: Ariston Publishers, 2004), 130. Originally published in English as *Sexual Secrets: The Alchemy of Ecstasy*.

21. Ibid., 124.

22. Alexander Lowen, *Bioenergetik für jeden: Das vollständige Übungshandbuch* [Bioenergetics for Everyone: The Complete Practice Guide] (Munich: Kirchhelm Publishers, 2003), 116. Originally published in English as *Bioenergetics*.

CHAPTER 2. ENERGETIC AND SPIRITUAL BASICS

1. Mantak Chia and Douglas Abrams Arava, *Öfter, länger, besser: Sextipps für den Mann* [More Frequent, Longer, Better: Sex Tips for Men] (Munich: Droemer Knaur Publishers, 2002), 41. Originally published in English as *The Multiorgasmic Man: Sexual Secrets That Every Man Should Know*.

2. Interview with Joseph Kramer, founder and director of the Body Electric School of Massage and Rebirthing, a school training physical therapists recognized by the state of California.

3. Ibid.

4. Ibid.

5. Ibid.

6. Interview with K. Ruby, sex researcher, coach, and sex educator.

7. Anna Trökes, "Hatha-Yoga," in *Der Weg des Yoga: Handbuch für Übende und Lehrende* [The Path of Yoga: Practical Guide for Students and Teachers] (Petersberg, Germany: Via Nova Publishers, 2000), 101.

8. Ibid.

9. Ibid.

CHAPTER 3. THE YONI MASSAGE

1. David Boadella, *Wilhelm Reich: Pionier des neuen Denkens—Eine Biographie* [Wilhelm Reich: A Biography of the Pioneer of New Thinking] (Munich: Droemer Knaur Publishers, 1998), 154–155.

Further Reading

Angier, Natalie. *Woman: An Intimate Geography*, reprint ed. New York: Anchor Books, 2000.

Boadella, David. *Wilhelm Reich: The Evolution of His Work*. New York: Penguin, 1988.

Castaneda, Carlos. *Magical Passes: The Practical Wisdom of the Shamans of Ancient Mexico*. New York: HarperPerennial, 1998.

Chia, Mantak. *Healing Love through the Tao: Cultivating Female Sexual Energy*. Rochester, Vt.: Destiny Books, 2005.

Chia, Mantak, and Douglas Abrams Arava. *The Multiorgasmic Man: Sexual Secrets That Every Man Should Know*. San Francisco: HarperSanFrancisco, 1997.

Douglas, Nik, and Penny Slinger. *Sexual Secrets: The Alchemy of Ecstasy*, twentieth anniversary edition. Rochester, Vt.: Destiny Books, 1999.

Jansen, Eva Rudy. Translated by Tony Langham. *The Book of Hindu Imagery: The Gods and Their Symbols*. Havelte, Holland: Binkey Kok Publications BV, 1993.

Lowen, Alexander. *Bioenergetics: The Revolutionary Therapy That Uses the Language of the Body to Heal the Problems of the Mind*. New York: Penguin/Arkana, 1994.

Northrup, Christiane, M.D. *Women's Bodies, Women's Wisdom: Creating Physical and Emotional Health and Healing*, 3rd. ed. New York: Bantam, 2006.

Walker, Barbara G. *The Woman's Encyclopedia of Myths and Secrets*. San Francisco: HarperSanFrancisco, 1983.

Wilber, Ken. *A Brief History of Everything*, 2nd ed. Boston: Shambhala, 2001.

Acknowledgments

I spent more than four years working on this book, with great engagement and a lot of effort, through highs and lows. This would not have been possible for me without the many people who supported, accompanied, and encouraged me in so many ways. My special thanks go to:

- My mother, Roswitha Riedl, who loves me unconditionally, accepts me as I am, and supports me wherever and however she can, and who is probably happier even than I that this book is finally finished.
- My father, Friedrich Riedl, who always respects my own ways, even if he is most often of a different opinion, and who through this shows me his love.
- My teacher and friend Maraya Haenen, who taught me to pray and gave me experiential answers to many of my life's questions. I learned so much from her that without her, I would be a different woman.
- My business partner and friend Gitta Arntzen, who is far more than an incredible support. I am thankful for every moment we have together, and for the fact that we are following a shared path and pursuing a shared vision through AnandaWave.
- My friend and first lecturer Constance Rinck, for her friendly presence and support despite too little time for this on my part, for the spontaneous walks, and for the "idea first and champagne after."
- My friend Karin Schell, for the sentence "Michaela, you definitely need an outline," for her cuddly friendship, for her humor, and for always being able to correct me.

- Monika Neumann, for her engagement and presence for AnandaWave and for the new opportunity of our encounter in a completely different way, for which I am very grateful.
- Susanne Dicken, of whom I thought often while writing this book.
- Dieter Grasbon, for his valuable corrections, for the "eagle's mouse" and the "doctor's view."
- Ella Gluck, for the drawings and the beautiful encounters over a "Koelsch."
- Andreas Skott, for the photos, for the cover of "Vaginam Tango," and for the many interesting conversations.
- Marion Schemann, for the statistics, even if they didn't fit into the book, for the interesting stories, and for olive oil and Francois Villon.
- Martina Weiser, Ananda (Art of Touch), Frankfurter Str. 40, 51065 Cologne, tel: +49-221-6086585, www.tantramassage.de, for the long path that we have walked together.
- Frank Fleuchaus and Bernd Eidenmueller, for the particularly sensual, focused, and professional twelve-hour photo session for this book, and for the idea to produce a DVD together with us.
- All the women who took part in my very intimate questionnaires and interviews, for their valuable statements and input and for the courage to open and show themselves.
- Tara-Maya Schmidt, Marion Usha Ajwani, Andrea, and Gitta Arntzen, for their work as photo models.
- Anna Raab, for joining me in ringing Joseph Kramer out of bed and for helping numerous times with the translations.
- Marion Usha Ajwani, for several suggestions for the subtitles, especially for "female lust to love."
- Antonia Alaris, for the wonderful poems that she allowed me to publish in the book, and for the poetry reading during the AnandaWave basic training, after I had received a yoni massage.
- Dr. Schmale, my primary care doctor, for his valuable interview, despite my being late.
- All "dragons" of the women's research group Dragon Trail: Bettina, Dorothee, Kali, Iris, Laura, Birgit, and Jutta, for the traces they left in this book.

- Annie Sprinkle, for the funny interview and her support.
- Hans Nietsch, my publisher, for the beautiful walks through Freiburg, and for having spent an entire weekend explaining to me the difference between preface and introduction, and for ensuring that the book turned out as well and beautifully as it did.
- All people, in particular the team of AnandaWave, who help Gitta and myself to realize the vision of AnandaWave.
- All readers—male and female—who let themselves be inspired by this book, and through that perhaps contribute to more understanding of our sexuality.

About the Author

⁓

Michaela Riedl, born in 1968 in Straubing, Bavaria, first studied music before learning tantric yoga. During these studies, she learned about erotic massage, tantric massage as taught by Andro of the Diamond Lotus Institute, as well as the yoni and lingam massages taught by Joseph Kramer and Annie Sprinkle, all of which contributed to her enthusiasm for tantric massage.

Touched and inspired by the healing effects of this massage work, she developed during the course of her experience an individual massage style and since 1997 has led her own massage seminars.

In cooperation with a partner, Michaela Riedl opened the tantric massage practice Ananda in October 1998, where she was responsible for guiding the program. During this time she attended further trainings and explored research about male and female sexuality. From these experiences, Michaela Riedl developed a newer version of classic tantra massage. In August 2005, Michaela Riedl and Gitta Arntzen opened a new space—AnandaWave, which offers modern tantric massage and seminars on "space for sensual experiences." The two owners offer people the opportunity to experience new forms of personal expression in the areas of sensuality, sexuality, and spirituality in individual ways.

The AnandaWave massage activates and energizes the entire body of the recipient in a dynamic and loving way. It awakens sexual energies and distributes these throughout the body. Special massage offerings focus on different aspects of personal healing.

The basis of the seminar offerings are the different massage workshops for women, men, and couples, as well as the training and advanced training (with certification) in AndandaWave tantric massage. These are complemented by different seminars related to bodywork, meditation, and personality development. Lectures on female and male sexuality, as well as demonstrations of AnandaWave massages, round out the program.

The holistic approach of AnandaWave is supported by sex and communication counseling for individuals and couples by Constanze Rinck, a systematic family therapist and communication trainer.

～

The book *Yoni Massage* by Michaela Riedl is an expression of her long experience in massage and seminar work, which she continues to refine together with Gitta Arntzen and the team at AnandaWave. Contact:

AnandaWave—Space for Sensual Experience
Michaela Riedl and Gitta Arntzen
Riehler Str. 23
50668 Cologne
Germany

Massage offerings: +49-221-1793511
Seminars and organization: +49-221-4208028

E-mail: info@ananda-wave.de
Websites: www.Ananda-Wave.de
           www.Tantramassagen.de

Index

Page numbers in *italics* refer to illustrations.